10 YEARS YOUNGER

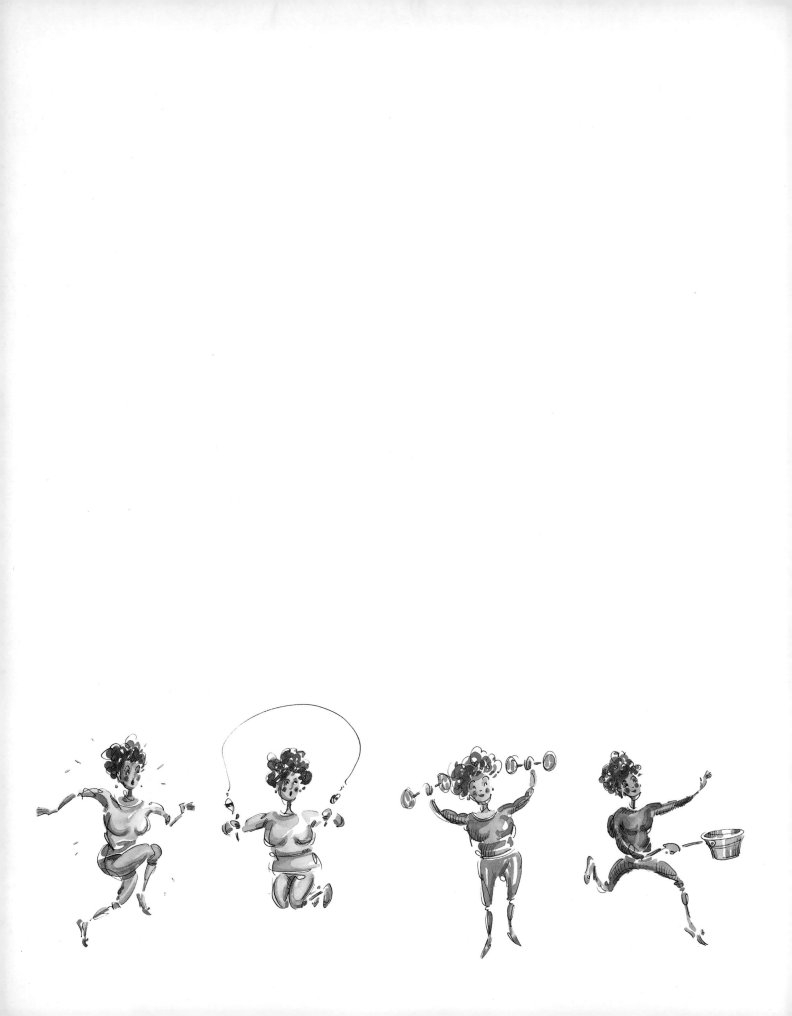

10 YEARS YOUNGER

Judith Wills

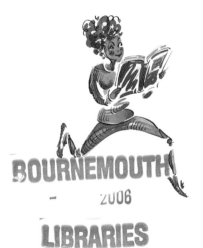

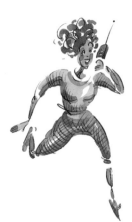

Quadrille

To Mother and Ann

The author and publishers would like to stress that this book expresses the well-informed opinions and experience of the author. Although we are confident that almost everyone will benefit from this book, we can in no way guarantee results of any kind. It would be advisable to seek your practitioner's advice and undergo a full physical examination prior to undertaking the programme.

The recipes in the book are for four people unless otherwise stated.

Both metric and imperial quantities are given.
Use either all metric or all imperial, as the two
are not necessarily interchangeable.

First published in 1997 by
Quadrille Publishing Ltd
Alhambra House
27-31 Charing Cross Road
London
WC2H 0LS

This paperback edition first published in 2005
10 9 8 7 6 5 4 3 2 1

Publishing Director: Anne Furniss
Art Director: Mary Evans
Project Editor: Lewis Esson
Design: Mary Staples
Editorial Assistant: Katherine Seely
Special Photography: Ian Hooton
Illustrations: Lynne Robinson and Julia Whatley
Picture Research: Nadine Bazar
Production: Candida Lane

Consultants
Wardrobe Styling: Ceril Campbell
Makeup: Celia Hunter
Hair Dressing: Paul Edmonds
Exercises: Louise Taylor

Cataloguing in Publication Data: a catalogue record for this book is
available from the British Library.

ISBN 1 84400 171 7
Printed in China

CONTENTS

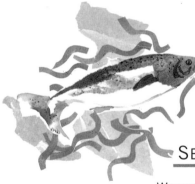

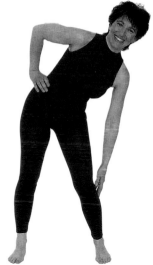

'I'm proud to be my age,' said a 45-year-old colleague of mine
when she heard that I was writing this book.
'Why do you want to encourage women to think they've got
to act and look like 25-year-olds?' she quite reasonably asked.

Well I don't. This book isn't about mimicking youth. I have no intention of helping you to look, or be, the same as you were then, or, indeed, of asking you to become a carbon copy of your teenage daughter. You don't want that; I don't want that.

But what I do set out to do is *improve* upon youth. To steal its assets, such as vitality and optimism, a fit body and glowing skin, and leave the rest very gladly behind.

I'm proud to say I'm 46. But I still enjoy it when I'm taken for 40, or even less. To me, it means I look after myself and that I care enough about life, and the people I love, to make an effort. And, of course, I very much hope that looking after myself means I will feel healthier and happier into a long and fulfilling old age!

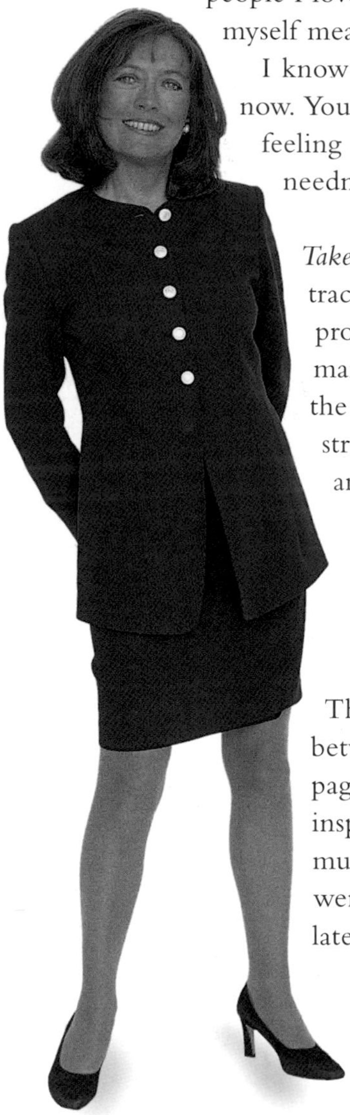

I know what you want, because it is what I want – to be, simply, my best for now. Your best, for now, is what this book is all about. Looking your best, feeling your best and enjoying your life. Why look old, why feel old when you needn't? Why get left behind?

Take Off Ten Years in Ten Weeks is the programme that helps get you back on track in every way - maybe, even, to find a new track. All I ask is that you promise to put yourself first, at least some of the time – something that many of you have *not* done in years. Women who have been adults through the 60s, 70s, 80s or 90s have, I believe, had the hardest, busiest, most stressful time of any generation of women, with choices, responsibilities, and problems that no other women have had to face.

Now is your time.
Time to get back in touch with yourself, your body and your needs.
And here is *your* book.

The 10-week course it contains has been tested by ordinary women aged between 35 and 57. You'll encounter several of them many times in the pages ahead as you work through the programme yourself. If you need inspiration or confirmation that you really can shed the years and feel so much better, look at the four participants who appear opposite (as they were at the start of the 10 weeks), then look at pages 138–41, 10 weeks later, and read the women's comments, too.

Ten weeks can change your life – if you let them!

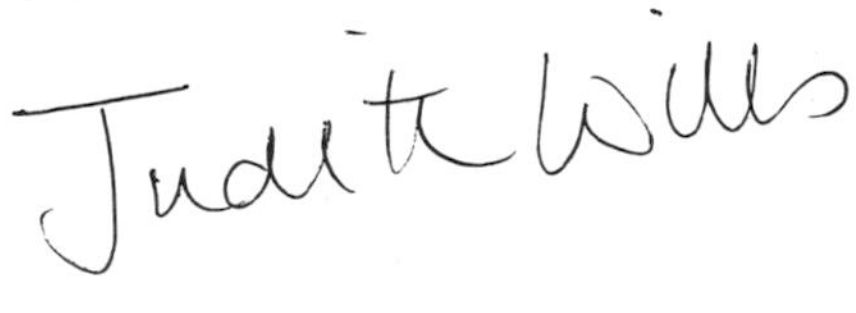

Judith Wills

MEET THE PARTICIPANTS

Now let me introduce you to our four main participants, Hilary, Sue, Pamela and Kay.
You'll be finding out much more about each of them, and how they are progressing,
as you work through the 10-week course.

Hilary Clarke

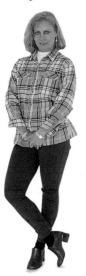

Sue Salkind

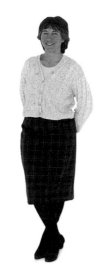

Pamela Newton

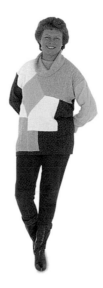

Kay Rainford

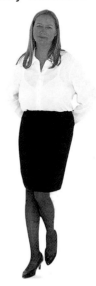

Hilary is a 43-year-old nursery nurse and married with two grown-up sons and a teenage daughter.

She has put on nearly a stone and a half since her 20's and has virtually given up buying new – clothes, 'because it is depressing when nothing looks right.'

A recent two-year college course made the problem worse – 'I couldn't resist the puddings in the college café!' and, although she goes to the swimming pool regularly, Hilary has difficulty sometimes in doing even one length.

'I get out of breath and feel dreadful – so I really want to get fitter.'

Hilary admits she hasn't changed her hairstyle or make-up in several years and is looking for new advice, as well as for some help with her problem skin, her lack of energy and stress levels.

Sue, 39, is a part-time GP, mother of two small daughters and is doing a course in acupuncture. Sue currently weighs nearly ten stone – 'Most of which appears to be around my tummy!' – and is finding it hard to motivate herself to exercise.

'As a doctor, I feel I should set a good example to my patients, but I'm afraid I don't. I am also something of a chocoholic and have got quite lazy in my eating habits. I really need you to give me the motivation I need to shape up and get fitter.'

Sue also admits that she is in dire need of a wardrobe re-think. 'I've bought hardly anything new since my girls were born and I've no confidence in shopping for myself. And I've never worn make-up, either.' I think it's time for a new look Sue . . .

Pamela is 57 and a housewife. She has two grown-up sons and is a grandmother. She lives with her husband, who is retired, and although she plays bowls and swims in the summer, two of her favourite hobbies – eating out and entertaining at home – have resulted in a weight gain of several stones over the years.

'I used to be a very slim 35-23-35, and it really depresses me when I catch a glimpse of myself unexpectedly. I love nice clothes but nothing looks good on me any more.'

Pamela is on HRT and feels this is going to stop her losing weight. 'I don't want to give up my lifestyle, either. I wonder what you are going to be able to do to help *me*!'

Kay, 49, is suffering a total loss of confidence, having been made redundant two years ago from her job as an administration assistant and having been rejected for hundreds of other posts. 'I feel my age is against me when applying for jobs,' she says. 'I think it would really help me to get somewhere if I look younger and feel better.' She is also recently divorced and living alone for the first time in her life.

At 10 stone, Kay, who is also on HRT after a hysterectomy the same year as her divorce and redundancy ('not a great year, really!'), is hardly overweight but she has never done any exercise at all and her body really is badly out of condition. 'I'm stuck in a time-warp as far as hair and clothes go, too. I feel the need of a complete overhaul!'

You will also be meeting Sal, Linda, and Angela during the programme, each of whom also
completed the 10-week course with our four participants above.

YOUR 10-WEEK TIMETABLE

Your schedule for the 10-week course begins opposite.
First read the notes below

THE COURSE IS DIVIDED INTO THREE SECTIONS.
THESE ARE:

MIRROR IMAGE
The Outer You

which deals with your body size and shape,
your skin, make-up, hair and wardrobe.

ENERGY SOURCES
The Vital You

which enhances and taps into your energy levels
in every possible way.

LIFE CHOICES
The Inner You

which helps you to explore possibilities and
re-think your life.

*Beginning of
Week*

1

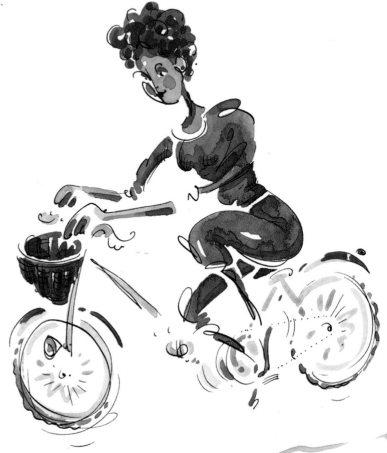

_____ *weight*

_____ *bust*

_____ *waist*

_____ *hips*

_____ *thighs*

_____ *energy levels*

_____ *BMI**

_____ *WHR**

COMMENTS

E ach of the three sections is divided into workshops, and we will be covering all these workshops in logical order over the next 10 weeks. Some workshops, such as your eating plan and the ShapeWise programmes, are ongoing throughout the 10 weeks and beyond. Others are short 'lessons' or assessments, which may take between 20 and 60 minutes of your time. I aim for the weekly time input on the course to be no more than 3 hours a week, plus occasional 'specials'.

All you need to do is follow the week-by-week timetable as laid out in the next 10 pages. Before you begin, read the introductions to each of the three sections (Mirror Image on page 19, Energy Sources on page 93 and Life Choices on page 118), which will give you a clear idea of what we're going to achieve.

At the start of each week, look at the workshops you're going to be covering in the week ahead, and schedule them into your week, using your own diary. Fill in all the blank weight, statistics, energy levels and comment boxes as you go along, for your own personal record.

Also, why not have a photo taken as you are now, then take one at the end of the 10 weeks just like our own participants did?

* see page 21

_____

weight

_____

bust

_____

waist

_____

hips

_____

thighs

_____

energy levels

COMMENTS

General notes:

- Fill in your starting weight and statistics opposite.

- Look at what we're going to be doing in the week ahead and the time it may take, and plan out your own schedule accordingly.

- Do the Assessments as early in the week as possible.

- Plan the most demanding workshops for your least busy days.

- Your personal eating plan will be ongoing through the weeks – take time to plan out your menus and shopping.

- Leave at least one clear day between each ShapeWise session to allow your body to recover.

WEEK ONE SCHEDULE

	workshop	page	time	notes
	Mirror Image			
I	**SIZING UP** – BODYWISE ASSESSMENT	20	*45 min*	
2	**PERSONAL EATING PLAN**	24	*Ongoing*	*but read through and familiarize*
3	**SHAPEWISE 1** – TOTAL TONE Session 1	36	*30 min*	*Familiarize*
3	**SHAPEWISE 1** – TOTAL TONE Session 2	36	*20 min*	*Your first real workout!*
3	**SHAPEWISE 1** – TOTAL TONE Session 3	36	*20 min*	
	Energy Sources			
II	**HEALTH CHECK**	94	*45 min*	*Make appointments as necessary*
I2	**TIME MANAGEMENT**	96	*30 min*	*Time allowed includes keeping daily diary*
	Life Choices			
I8	**NETWORKING**	119	*30 min*	*Read through; decide what is relevant to you; make a plan.*

End of Week

2

weight

bust

waist

hips

thighs

energy levels

COMMENTS

WEEK TWO SCHEDULE

	workshop	page	time	notes
	Mirror Image			
2	**PERSONAL EATING PLAN**	24	Ongoing	
3	**SHAPEWISE** – TOTAL TONE Session 1	36	*20 min*	
3	**SHAPEWISE** – TOTAL TONE Session 2	36	*20 min*	
3	**SHAPEWISE** – TOTAL TONE Session 3	36	*20 min*	
5	**BARE ESSENTIALS**	52	*20 min*	*Read through.*
5	**BARE ESSENTIALS**	52	*15 min*	*Shop for items needed when convenient.*
	Energy Sources			
12	**TIME MANAGEMENT**	96	*20 min*	*How much time can you save? Analyse your week I daily diary using guidelines in workshop. Write down your intentions.*
14	**IMPROVE YOUR STAMINA**	105	*30 min*	*Read through and do the Measured Mile Test.*
14	**IMPROVE YOUR STAMINA**	105	*20 min*	*Start on Stage One.*
	Life Choices			
19	**EDUCATION**	122	*45 min*	*Read through; make your own plans.*

WEEK THREE SCHEDULE

workshop		page	time	notes
	Mirror Image			
2	**PERSONAL EATING PLAN**	24	*Ongoing*	
3	**SHAPEWISE 1** – TOTAL TONE Session 1	36	*20 min*	
3	**SHAPEWISE 1** – TOTAL TONE Session 2	36	*20 min*	
3	**SHAPEWISE 1** – TOTAL TONE Session 3	36	*20 min*	
4	**SHAPEWISE 2** – BODY ALIGNMENT	48	*20 min*	*Read through and do Mirror Test. Familiarize yourself with exercises.*
5	**BARE ESSENTIALS** – 20-minute Facial	56	*20 min*	*Ideal time for this is after a bath.*
	Energy Sources			
14	**STAMINA** – Session 1	105	*20 min*	
14	**STAMINA** – Session 2	105	*20 min*	
14	**STAMINA** – Mind Games	107	*15 min*	*Try this panel as often as you like.*
	Life Choices			
20	**EXPLORATION**	124	*20 min*	

End of Week

3

_____
weight

_____
bust

_____
waist

_____
hips

_____
thighs

_____
energy levels

COMMENTS

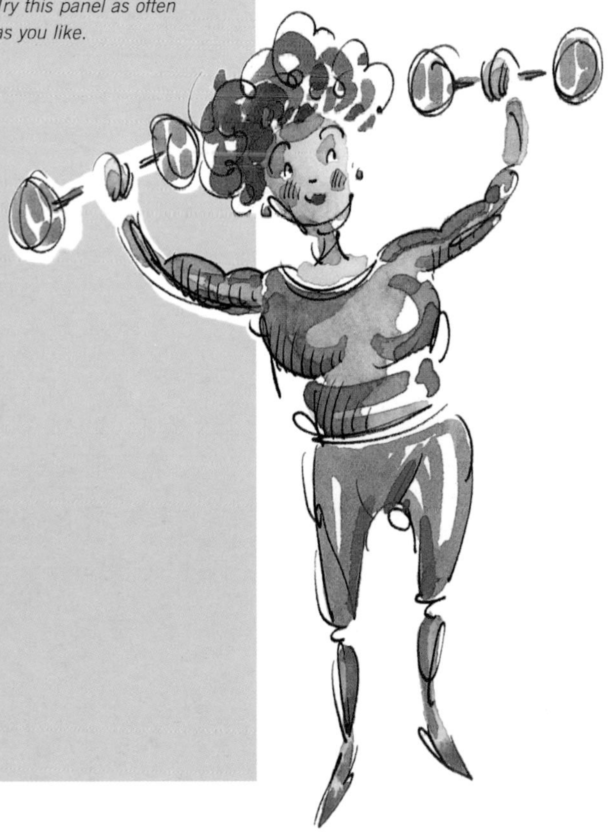

End of Week

4

_____
weight

_____
bust

_____
waist

_____
hips

_____
thighs

_____
energy levels

COMMENTS

WEEK FOUR SCHEDULE

	workshop	page	time	notes
	Mirror Image			
2	**PERSONAL EATING PLAN**	24	*Ongoing*	
3	**SHAPEWISE 1**– TOTAL TONE Session 1	36	*20 min*	
3	**SHAPEWISE 1**– TOTAL TONE Session 2	36	*20 min*	
3	**SHAPEWISE 1**– TOTAL TONE Session 3	36	*20 min*	
4	**SHAPEWISE 2** – BODY ALIGNMENT	48	*5 min*	*Optional*
5	**BARE ESSENTIALS** – Almost-free Facelift	58	*15 min*	*Try to do these exercises for 2-3 minutes twice a day through the programme*
	Energy Sources			
14	**STAMINA** – Session 1	105	*20 min*	
14	**STAMINA** – Session 2	105	*20 min*	
14	**STAMINA** – Session 3	105	*20 min*	
15	**LEARN TO RELAX**	108	*30 min*	*Read through and put into context of your own life.*
	Life Choices			
21	**SOCIABILITY** – FRIENDS	126	*15 min*	

WEEK FIVE SCHEDULE

workshops	page	time	notes
Mirror Image			
2 PERSONAL EATING PLAN	24	*Ongoing*	
3 SHAPEWISE 1– TOTAL TONE Session 1	36	*20 min*	
3 SHAPEWISE 1 – TOTAL TONE Session 2	36	*20 min*	
3 SHAPEWISE 1 – TOTAL TONE Session 3	36	*20 min*	
4 SHAPEWISE 2 – BODY ALIGNMENT	48	*5 min*	*Optional*
6 MAKE-UP MAGIC	58	*30 min*	*Read through and study photos and ideas.*
Energy Sources			
14 STAMINA – Session 1	105	*20 min*	
14 STAMINA – Session 2	105	*20 min*	
14 STAMINA – Session 3	105	*20 min*	
15 LEARN TO RELAX – SELF-MASSAGE	110	*10 min*	
Life Choices			
21 SOCIABILITY – FAMILY MATTERS	129	*30 min*	

_____
weight

_____
bust

_____
waist

_____
hips

_____
thighs

_____
energy levels

COMMENTS

End of Week

6

weight	
bust	
waist	
hips	
thighs	
energy levels	

COMMENTS

WEEK SIX SCHEDULE

	workshop	page	time	notes
	Mirror Image			
2	**PERSONAL EATING PLAN**	24	*Ongoing*	
3	**SHAPEWISE 1** – TOTAL TONE Session 1	36	*20 min*	
3	**SHAPEWISE 1** – TOTAL TONE Session 2	36	*20 min*	
3	**SHAPEWISE 1** – TOTAL TONE Session 3	36	*20 min*	
4	**SHAPEWISE 2** – BODY ALIGNMENT	48	*5 min*	*Optional*
6	**MAKE-UP MAGIC**	58	*1 hour*	*Go through your own make-up bag and decide what you need to throw away/buy. Buy what you need, taking advantage of department store make-overs.*
	Energy Sources			
14	**STAMINA** – Session 1	105	*20 min+*	*Increase your time when ready.*
14	**STAMINA** – Session 2	105	*20 min+*	
14	**STAMINA** – Session 3	105	*20 min+*	
16	**DEEP SLEEP**	112	*15 min*	*Optional for insomnia – read through and see what you would like to try.*
	Life Choices			
22	**RELATIONSHIPS 1**	130	*30 min*	*For women already in a relationship.*
	or			
23	**RELATIONSHIPS 2**	132	*30 min*	*For women seeking a relationship.*

WEEK SEVEN SCHEDULE

	workshop	page	time	notes
	Mirror Image			
2	**PERSONAL EATING PLAN**	24	*Ongoing*	*Don't forget – once you reach target weight, move to the Zest Plan on page 103.*
3	**SHAPEWISE 1** – TOTAL TONE Session 1	36	*20 min*	
3	**SHAPEWISE 1** – TOTAL TONE Session 2	36	*20 min*	
3	**SHAPEWISE 1** – TOTAL TONE Session 3	36	*20 min*	
4	**SHAPEWISE 2** – BODY ALIGNMENT	48	*5 min*	*Optional – if you have poor posture you will benefit from daily Shapewise 2 sessions.*
6	**MAKE-UP MAGIC**	58	*20 min*	*Give yourself a new make-up look using your new cosmetics, and the information in the workshop for guidance.*
7	**HAIR FLAIR 1** – SUPERSTYLES	66	*20 min+*	
	Energy Sources			
14	**STAMINA** – Session 1	105	*20 min+*	
14	**STAMINA** – Session 2	105	*20 min+*	
14	**STAMINA** – Session 3	105	*20 min+*	
17	**ZAPPING THE NEGATIVES**	115	*20 min*	
	Life Choices			
24	**PURE PLEASURE**	136	*20 min*	

weight

bust

waist

hips

thighs

energy levels

COMMENTS

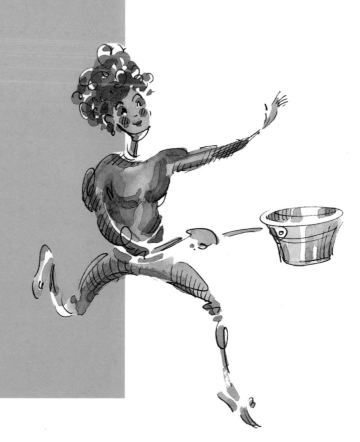

End of Week

8

_____
weight
_____
bust
_____
waist
_____
hips
_____
thighs
_____
energy levels

COMMENTS

WEEK EIGHT SCHEDULE

workshop		page	time	notes
	Mirror Image			
2	**PERSONAL EATING PLAN**	24	*Ongoing*	
3	**SHAPEWISE 1** – TOTAL TONE Session 1	36	*20 min*	
3	**SHAPEWISE 1** – TOTAL TONE Session 2	36	*20 min*	
3	**SHAPEWISE 1** – TOTAL TONE Session 3	36	*20 min*	
4	**SHAPEWISE 2** – BODY ALIGNMENT	48	*5 min*	
7	**HAIR FLAIR 1** – SUPERSTYLES *special* – Salon Hair-cut	68	*1 hour+*	
8	**HAIR FLAIR 2** – COLOUR AND CONDITION	70	*15 min*	
9	**STYLE ASSESSMENT 1** – FINDING YOUR OWN STYLE	76	*20 min+*	
	Energy Sources			
14	**STAMINA** – Session 1	105	*20 min+*	
14	**STAMINA** – Session 2	105	*20 min+*	
14	**STAMINA** – Session 3	105	*20 min+*	
12	**TIME MANAGEMENT**	96		
15	**LEARN TO RELAX**	108	*30 min*	
16	**DEEP SLEEP**	112		
17	**ZAPPING THE NEGATIVES**	115		
	Life Choices			
18	**NETWORKING**	119	*20 min*	
19	**EDUCATION**	122	*20 min*	

WEEK NINE SCHEDULE

workshop	page	time	notes
Mirror Image			
2 PERSONAL EATING PLAN	24	*Ongoing*	
3 SHAPEWISE 1 – TOTAL TONE Session 1	36	*20 min*	
3 SHAPEWISE 1 – TOTAL TONE Session 2	36	*20 min*	
3 SHAPEWISE 1 – TOTAL TONE Session 3	36	*20 min*	
4 SHAPEWISE 2 – BODY ALIGNMENT	48	*5 min*	*Optional*
9 STYLE ASSESSMENT 1 – WARDROBE WORKOUT	85	*1 hour*	*Sort out your wardrobe following the guidelines in part one of the box on page 85.*
10 STYLE ASSESSMENT 2 – DRESSING FOR YOUR SHAPE	86	*1 hour*	*Read the workshop and assess your pared-down wardrobe for 'shape suitability'. Decide what, if anything, you need to buy.*
Energy Sources			
14 STAMINA – Session 1	105	*20 min+*	
14 STAMINA – Session 2	105	*20 min+*	
14 STAMINA – Session 3	105	*20 min+*	
Life Choices			
20 EXPLORATION	124	*20 min*	*Re-read these two workshops and assess your own progress. Make notes for the future.*
21 SOCIABILITY	126	*20 min*	

---
weight

---
bust

---
waist

---
hips

---
thighs

---
energy levels

COMMENTS

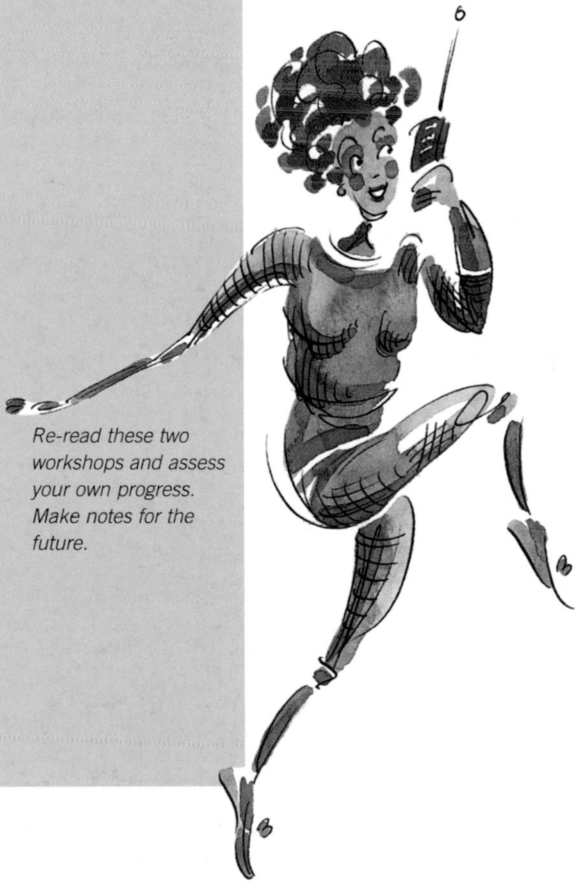

End of Week

10

weight
bust
waist
hips
thighs
energy levels
BMI *
WHR *
COMMENTS

WEEK TEN SCHEDULE

	workshop	page	time	notes
	Mirror Image			
1	**BODY ASSESSMENTS**	20	*15 min*	*Re-assess your BMI, WHR, your target weight and your shape in the mirror; write your comments.*
2	**PERSONAL EATING PLAN**	24	*Ongoing*	
3	**SHAPEWISE 1** – TOTAL TONE Session 1	36	*20 min*	
3	**SHAPEWISE 1** – TOTAL TONE Session 2	36	*20 min*	
3	**SHAPEWISE 1** – TOTAL TONE Session 3	36	*20 min*	
4	**SHAPEWISE 2** – BODY ALIGNMENT	48	*5 min*	*Optional*
8	**HAIR FLAIR 2** – COLOUR & CONDITION	70	*1-2 hours*	*Optional – if you're not sure about changing colour, ask the head colourist at your salon.*
9	**STYLE ASSESSMENT 1** – SHOPPING TRIP	85	*half day+*	*Have fun! Choose some new clothes following the guidelines in Wardrobe Revamp, part 2.*
	Energy Sources			
11	**HEALTH CHECK**	94	*1 hour*	*Re-read this workshop and reassess your health.*
14	**STAMINA** – SESSION 1	105	*20 min+*	
14	**STAMINA** – SESSION 2	105	*20 min+*	
14	**STAMINA** – SESSION 3	105	*20 min+*	
	Life Choices			
22	**RELATIONSHIPS 1** *or*	130	*20 min*	*Re-read these two workshops and note the improvements you've made.*
23	**RELATIONSHIPS 2**	132		
24	**PURE PLEASURE**	136		

Congratulations!

You have completed the 10-week course.

Check out your final weight and statistics; assess how you feel.

Take that photo of yourself with your new hair and make-up, wearing some new clothes and a big smile.

Compare it with how you looked 10 weeks ago; how you looked 10 years ago.

Please write and let me know your verdict and send me those photos!

* see page 21

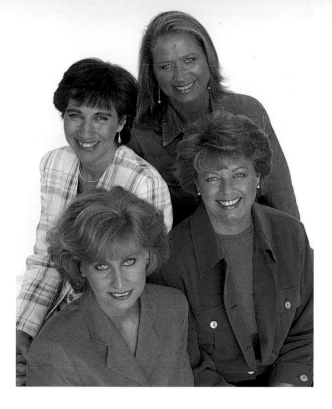

MIRROR IMAGE

The Outer You

How long since you took a good look in the mirror? How long since you liked what you saw? In fact – how long since you noticed how you really look? It can become very easy to get used to extra pounds or stones; flabbiness where your flesh used to be firm. 'I'm getting older – I might as well accept it' goes the familiar cry.

No. No, no, NO! The Mirror Image workshops will help you to see yourself afresh and to make objective decisions about what you can change, what those changes should be, and how to go about them. It is NEVER too late to re-style your body and your looks and shed the years. Your body doesn't have to succumb to middle-aged spread.

Research reveals that exercise in mid-life shows just as quick results as in your 20s. And losing weight, while a slower process than when you are young, is not as impossible a task as you may have been led to believe!

In the same way, old familiar hair, make-up and style looks may be comforting and easy – but it's a very rare woman indeed who can look her best with the same make-up, hair and wardrobe she had 10 – even 5 – years ago.

Whether you just need updating, or even gave up the ghost completely years ago and now go make-up free with your hair pulled back and always live in leggings and a baggy jumper – you'll find the answers here. Your body deserves some attention. Now is the time to give it. Here is the place.

*F*ew women approaching – or in – their mid years have a body as slim or firm
as it was in their teens and twenties. In Workshop 1, we assess your physical
appearance and make realistic decisions about just how much you can turn back time.

WORKSHOP 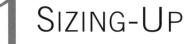 SIZING-UP

Your Weight

One of the most common physical
signs of ageing is weight gain. So
many of us experience this that the
dreaded 'middle-age spread' is
thought of as natural and
inevitable. The woman of 40
who can still fit into the
wedding dress she wore at 20
is seen as something of a
phenomenon. And the truth
is that to stay as slim as you were
in your teens and 20s, you do need to
eat less than you did then (more on the
reasons for this is in Workshop 2).

However, don't be too envious of those few
skinny women, because all the latest research
shows that putting on a little weight as we get
older is probably a good thing, and that being thin
and living on a meagre diet is not. One of the
main consequences of thinness is an increased likelihood of osteoporosis, which any sensible woman
would prefer to avoid if possible. Also, there is
evidence that menopausal symptoms may be more
severe in thin women. And, should you – like most
of us – fear wrinkles as much as being fat, a thin face
is much more likely to show noticeable wrinkles than
one 'plumped up' by a small layer of fat.

No, what you want to achieve is BALANCE – a
weight that is, perhaps, up to a stone heavier than that
you were at 20 (if you were slim then), but not much
more. Too much fat is ageing and even more bad for
your health than being too thin. A good rule of
thumb for how much weight gain is acceptable for
you is to put on no more than 3-4 pounds for
every decade you are over 25. So if you were, say,

> ### Can I lose weight if I'm on HRT?
>
> If you are overweight and on HRT –
> yes, you can slim. Again, there is no
> scientific evidence that shows you have to
> gain weight with HRT – though many women
> do. And, as our guinea pig Pamela (who is on
> HRT) proves, it is not as hard as you might
> think to lose that weight. But the rules for
> weight loss apply even more strongly if you
> are on HRT. Exercise! Don't aim too low! Don't
> expect fast loss!

9 stones in your early 20s, by 35 a weight of 9
stone 4 lb would be fine, by 45 a reasonable
weight is 9 stone 8 lb and by 55 about 9 stone 12
lb would be good going. Work this scale out now
for yourself.

If you are within this target for your age, my
advice is that you don't need to slim – use the
Zest Eating Plans on page 103 rather than the
slimming diet in Workshop 2, and if you still feel
you are fat, the shape assessment that follows will
probably reveal that all you need is better muscle
tone. However, if you have put on more than
this 'ideal gain', you probably would look better
and younger for shedding some weight.

Let's check you out further now,
then, by working out your
Body Mass Index – the
modern equivalent of the
height/weight charts – to
see just how overweight
you are.

ASSESSING YOUR WEIGHT AND SHAPE

The Body Mass Index

This involves using a calculator, so find yours and then here's what you do.

- **Start with your current weight in kilograms.**
  (To convert pounds into kilograms, divide by 2.2)

- **Convert your height into metres.**
  (To convert inches into metres, multiply by 0.025)

- **Square your height.**

- **Now finally divide your weight by your squared height.**

- **THE ANSWER IS YOUR BMI.**

Example:
You weigh 10 stone 10 lb.
(150 lb ÷ 2.2 equals **68 kg**).

You are 5 ft 5 in tall
(65 in x 0.025 equals **1.62 metres**).

Your height squared
(1.62 x 1.62 is **2.62**).

Your BMI (**68** divided by **2.62** is **25.95**).
Round this up to 26.

The international classification for BMIs is:

Below 20	*Underweight.*
20–25	*Acceptable weight range.*
25–30	*Overweight.*
30–40	*Obese (extremely overweight)*
Over 40	*Very obese (life-threateningly obese)*

Work out your own BMI here:

Current weight in kg ....

Height in metres ....

Height squared ....

Weight divided by height squared ....
Rounded up or down to the nearest half

MY BMI is......................................

Interpreting the results:

20 or below:
You should consider putting on some weight to bring your BMI between 20 and 25.

Over 30:
You are definitely overweight and you need to slim. Start tomorrow. Workshop 2 will help you do that.

25 – 30:
You probably need to slim – the nearer to 30 you are, the higher that likelihood goes. If your BMI is over 25 – but not much over – *here are some points to bear in mind* –

- If your weight is concentrated around your middle, but you have slim arms and legs, you are likely to need to slim.

- If you have heavy arms and legs, perhaps a large bust, but a reasonably slim midriff, you may not need to slim. I have seen two women of the same weight and height – one with a 33-inch waist, the other with a 28-inch waist. I advised the large-waisted woman to slim, but not the other. The reason an 'apple-shaped' woman should slim is that the apple-shape is linked with heart disease more than the classic female 'pear shape'. And as women enter their menopause years they are more predisposed to develop an 'apple shape', probably because of the hormonal changes that happen then.

If you are not sure if you have the 'apple shape', an easy test is to divide your waist measurement by your hip measurement. If the resulting figure is over 0.80, you are an 'apple'.

This figure is your Waist-to-Hip Ratio.

20 – 25:
If you are within the acceptable weight range and haven't put on more than the 'ideal gain' explained opposite since your 20's, then you don't need to slim. If you think you do, exercise is probably your answer. If your BMI is 20-25 and you HAVE put on more than the 'ideal gain' per decade, maybe you could do with losing a little, *but only if:*

- Your BMI is nearer 25 than 20 and

- Your Waist-to-Hip Ratio (explained above) is 0.80 or more.

To Sum Up:

- You want to be a healthy weight, not skinny.

- A healthy size can vary from person to person but, in general, it is healthier to be a large 'pear' than an 'apple'.

- If you are overweight, it is better to lose a sensible amount and keep it off, than it is to try to lose a lot and keep 'yo-yoing'.

HEIGHT WEIGHT CONVERSION CHART

14 pounds (lb) = 1 stone
2.205 pounds = 1 kilogramme (kg)

12 inches = 1 foot
1 inch = 2.5 centimetres
40 inches = 1 metre

Have years of yo-yo dieting ruined my metabolism?

It is a popular myth that if, as many women now in their 30s, 40s and 50s did, you spend years on and off diets, with weight going then returning, your metabolism is affected so that eventually you can no longer lose weight, however much you reduce your food intake. This, you will be pleased to hear, is not true. Researchers at the Dunn Nutrition Unit, the internationally respected UK obesity research centre in Cambridge have found no evidence of metabolism affected in this way in scientifically-conducted trials of yo-yo dieters. What does happen is that as most people get older, they take less exercise, their muscle mass diminishes and, as muscle uses up more calories than other body tissue, the body's ability to burn calories, and therefore shed weight (or stay slim) diminishes too. And, if you've yo-yo'd for years, you are psychologically programmed to believe you are going to fail.

So the rules for successful weight loss – and keeping it off – as you get older are:

• It's vital to exercise.

• It's vital not to aim for too low a weight.

• It's vital to accept a slow or steady weight-loss rather than a rapid one.

• And, of course, it is vital to eat a healthy diet while slimming – which is what you will find in the next workshop.

Your Shape

So – you are going to lose weight, if necessary, to get down to a size that is right for you now. But what about your body SHAPE? By their late 30s and beyond, many women have lumps and bumps, saggy, baggy or droopy bits on their bodies that aren't there just because of fat. They are there due to lack of body tone and poor posture. You don't have to put up with them. *Take Off 10 Years in 10 Weeks* is here to help. But first let's take the shape test.

THE SHAPE TEST

Stand in front of a full-length mirror with no clothing on (make it a warm room, then!), with this book and a pen to hand and complete the sections below.

1. Look at your body from top to toe and write down all the good things about it; all the things you like. *Yes – you can find some.* Everyone has good points. Don't be shy – no-one else is going to see this. *Write them here, or if you prefer, in a notebook.*

2. Check out the things you can't alter. We have to be realistic. You can't alter (except maybe through surgery): length of limbs, width of pelvis (hip bone structure), basic bone structure, shape of head, genetic tendency to a particular body shape – e.g. pear. You can improve your basic shape, but not turn yourself into your genetic opposite. For example, if you are a 'pear' with wide hips and big thighs with a small upper body and bust, you can slim your hips and thighs somewhat and firm them up, and develop your upper body through exercise, but you can't get narrow hips and long skinny legs like Elle McPherson.

Genetic tendency to a particular body-type.
There are three classifications of type:
Ectomorph (long and skinny);
Endomorph (curvy and with a tendency to put on body fat easily)
Mesomorph (strong and muscular, sporty).

Most people have one of those three types dominant, with a little of one or even both of the others mixed in. *See if you can spot your dominant type.*

Ectomorphs find it hard to put on weight when young, but may when they get older; **endomorphs** are always having to watch what they eat to keep their weight down, and **mesomorphs** can stay slim and build muscle easily but need plenty of physical activity. If your natural tendency is to, say, ectomorph, you will not be being realistic if your intention is to work out and build big muscles; be happy with a fit lean body. Be sensible.
Write down what your basic body type is here:

So there are things you can't change. That doesn't matter. This is your body, accept those things you can't alter and learn to like – or even love – the uniqueness of your body. In fact, go back and add that to your list of things you like about your body – it is unique. I am unique!

3. Find out the things you can change. (If you are more than a little overweight, you may find it hard to differentiate between body fat and lack of body tone, but if you're not sure about any of the items below, tick 'yes'.)

Here is a list of body symptoms that we can alter through exercise, from top to toe. Go through the list and tick any of them that apply to you.

Chin	❏ *double*
	❏ *saggy*
Neck	❏ *sunk into shoulders, seems too short*
Shoulders front on	❏ *very sloping, weak*
side on	❏ *rounded/hunched*
Upper arms	❏ *saggy, flabby underneath* (lift them out to sides and shake)
Bust	❏ *droopy*
Waist	❏ *thick*
Stomach side on	❏ *protruding*
Hips	❏ *flabby, love handles*
Bottom	❏ *flat*
	❏ *spread*
	❏ *droopy*
Thighs	❏ *spread*
Knees	❏ *fat*
Calves	❏ *lack definition*
Ankles	❏ *thick*
Feet	❏ *flat*

Right! Don't be disheartened if you ticked more than a few. It's almost as easy to shape up every bit of you as it is to shape up one bit! Workshops 3 and 4 and, to a lesser extent, workshop 13 will transform you over the weeks ahead.

4. Now, one last thing. Take a photo of yourself (OK, you can put a swimsuit on if you like!), front on and side on. You'll want to look back at it in 10 weeks' time and see just HOW much you've changed.

OUR PARTICIPANTS ASSESSED

Hilary has put on about 19 pounds since her 20s, has a BMI slightly over the ideal band of 20-25 with the surplus fat distributed quite evenly over her waist, hips, bottom and thighs. I am going to set her target weight at around 9 stone 7 lb which will bring her BMI down to just over 23, and I would like to see her lose an inch or two from around her waist – she wants to lose it from her butt, hips, thighs and knees!

'I hate my knees – they are too fat to get into a pair of tapered trousers I have!' Hilary swims regularly, but finds it hard going, and does no other exercise. The toning routine should firm her up all over and our stamina workshop (Workshop 14, page 105) will certainly increase her aerobic fitness.

HILARY, 43
Bust 35 in
Waist 29½ in
Hips 37¼ in
Thighs 23 in
BMI 25.5
Waist-to-hip ratio .79
Weight 10 stone 5 lb
Height 5 ft 4½ in
General body tone 'Soft' and lacking in tone all over
Fitness level Slightly fit

Sue is just inside the top of the ideal BMI range and her waist-to-hip ratio is fine, but she felt she did want to lose a few pounds. *'I know my WHR seems OK, but the weight HAS mostly gone on around my tummy and, as I'm short-waisted, it looks even worse.'* So we applied the 'weight gain per decade' criterion described earlier. In her mid 20s, Sue was 8½ stone. By nearing 40, then, a reasonable normal weight gain would be 7 pounds, so the minimum she should aim to be now is 9 stone. However I thought that might be unnecessarily low, so set Sue's target at 9 stone 2 lb.

She will do plenty of abdominal exercise for waist and stomach as well as the total tone routine and, as she enjoys aerobic classes will work out to a videotape our trainer Louise has made for our participants in order to improve her fitness, as well as fitting in tennis, walking and a session on a Healthrider when she can.

SUE, 39
Bust 35½ in
Waist 29½ in
Hips 39½ in
Thighs 22¼ in
BMI 24.7
Waist-to-hip ratio .75
Weight 9 stone 13 lb
Height 5 ft 4 in
General body tone Legs not too bad; abdomen, bottom, back and arms quite poor
Fitness level Slightly fit

Pamela is slightly overweight according to the BMI, and her WHR is also poor – she's a classic 'apple', with most of her surplus weight round her middle and with slim arms and legs. Add to that the fact that when she was in her 20s she weighed a mere 7½ stone, and has a tiny bone structure, and we agreed that Pamela should aim to lose around a stone, bringing her BMI down to approximately 23, a good weight IF she can reduce her waist and build a little muscle tone there, and on her limbs.

Although Pam plays bowls every week and sometimes does a little gentle swimming and walking, none of this is enough to keep her toned or aerobically fit, or to keep her bone density. We prescribed for her regular walking as detailed in the Stamina Workshop, as well as Louise's aerobic tape and we have given Pam a cross-trainer (a mini trampoline) to work out on when she gets odd spare moments at home. This is low-impact and very good for older women.

PAMELA, 57
Bust 38½ in
Waist 34½ in
Hips 40 in
Thighs 21½ in
BMI 25.3
Waist-to-hip ratio .86
Weight 10 stone 7 lb
Height 5 ft 5 in
General body tone Poor, especially abdomen, obliques, arms and legs
Fitness level Very unfit

Kay, on paper, is an ideal weight, but she needs to redistribute this weight in order to look really good. She is a typical case of someone who is slim, but has a low percentage of lean body tissue (muscle) and a high percentage of body fat. Her bust, waist and abdomen carry most of this fat, and she may need to lose a few pounds to get her WHR down to below .80 and to get her top half more in proportion. Her limbs, particularly her legs, are slim but with little muscle definition, so she needs to work hard on her exercise to build muscle up in these areas. Her bust will also look less 'droopy' if she tones up her pectorals and shoulders.

Kay has never taken any toning or aerobic exercise, so we need to build her stamina. At 49 and smoking 20 cigarettes a day, Kay is worried that this is all going to be an impossible task – but we have assured her that if she eats sensibly, begins exercise gently and builds up to regular long sessions of walking, aerobics and toning, as well as frequent sessions on her Healthrider, she will see good results.

KAY, 49
Bust 39½ in
Waist 32 in
Hips 38½ in
Thighs 17¼ in
BMI 22.7
Waist-to-hip ratio .83
Weight 10 stone
Height 5 ft 7 in
General body tone Poor with weak abdominals, shoulders, arms and legs
Fitness level Very unfit

*S*o you need to lose some weight – and you have ten weeks in which to do it. What can you expect to achieve? Following the plan in the pages that follow, you will lose up to 1½ stones without fuss. Shedding that fat is pain-free, with the delicious meals and recipes in the SizeWise Eating Plan (page 26). However, if you want to put ON weight – or simply maintain your existing weight – turn to the Eating for Energy Workshop 13 (page 100) where you'll find all the information you need on eating to shed the YEARS instead.

WORKSHOP 2 YOUR PERSONAL EATING PLAN

If your idea of a diet is deprivation and misery then think again. You can – indeed, you should – eat plenty while you lose those unwanted pounds of fat that have somehow accumulated over the years. But what you need to do is start thinking of food as fuel: good fuel for your body. Give your body good-quality fuel and the minimum of rubbish, and it will respond by shedding weight without leaving you feeling tired, hungry or depressed. A good diet – whether for slimming or not – can help you to feel better and look better too.

Good nutritious food is one of the keys to youthful looks and vitality. The right diet can improve the condition and appearance of your skin, hair, eyes and gums; and can help protect your health in many ways. You'll find more about healthy eating in Workshop 13 (page 100) but, for now, be assured that the diet you'll find here is a healthy weight-loss diet including all the nutrients your body needs for good health and well-being while you reshape your body.

The SizeWise Eating Plan consists of a 'flying-start' first week, followed by nine weeks of multi-choice meals, allowing you to eat to suit your lifestyle and preferences. If you reach your target weight before the 10 weeks are up, simply move to the plan in Workshop 13. If you finish the 10 weeks and still have more to lose, just carry on.

Before you begin, remember that slimming is not just about choosing the right foods, but also about having the right attitude. So do first read the eating tips that follow.

Eating Tips and Information

1. The key to any successful slimming diet is to get in touch with your appetite: which means learning to recognize hunger for what it is; and every other reason to eat for what IT is – a wrong reason! Beginning today, try these methods to reduce – drastically – the number of times in a day that you eat for the wrong reasons:

Every time you are about to eat something, say, 'Do I really need this? Am I truly hungry?' A lot of the time you will find yourself eating for other reasons—especially if the food or snack (or drink) in front of you is something fatty, sugary or low in nutrients (a 'rubbish' food). You may be bored or miserable, or maybe you're tempted to eat a leftover food as you load the dishes. If you can resist food your body doesn't need for fuel, you're well on the way to winning. If you can't resist, don't feel guilty – after all, you have years of habits to 'unlearn', and every small victory, will – eventually – turn into a new habit for life.

When serving food, pay attention to your portion sizes. We often pile much more on our plates than we really need. If you still genuinely do need more food when the plate is empty, you can always have a bit more. If it is on the plate, however, the natural inclination is to eat it, even if you are quite satisfied. Not necessarily through greed – either we just don't think, or we've had years of being told that leaving food is wasteful. It isn't necessary to measure out all your food, even on the SizeWise plan, but if you tend towards putting slightly less on the plate than you think you'll want (with the exception of the 'unlimited' foods we'll discuss later) and then you eat SLOWLY, you will often find you can cut portion sizes of the calorie-rich foods by a quarter or more.

When you are eating, as you get towards the end of your meal, learn to listen to your body. Have you had enough, even though there IS some left? Learn to stop eating when you are satisfied – again, slow eating will help you here. If you habitually have food left on the plate, you will know that you should be giving yourself smaller portions.

Always remember the 'good fuel' rule. When you ARE hungry, never feel guilty for eating 'good fuel'. This means fresh, natural, unadulterated foods such as raw salad items, lightly cooked vegetables, fruits of all kinds, lean protein, natural carbohydrates such as wholegrain breads, rice, pasta, and pulses. Good fuel is also, in moderation, fresh nuts and seeds, pure vegetable oils and oily fishes. (You'll learn more about good fuel in Workshop 13). Bad fuel is all kinds of highly processed items, high on calories, sugar and/or fat, but low on nutrients. Bad fuel is also TOO MUCH of certain foods that are OK eaten occasionally. For instance, Cheddar cheese contains protein, calcium and vitamins, but because it is high in saturated fat – and also in calories – a lot of it isn't good for your body or your slimming diet. The SizeWise plan provides you with a diet that is very high in good fuel and low on poor fuel.

2. Eat regularly – from when you wake up to when you have your evening meal, don't allow more than three hours to go by without eating something. Yes, this IS a diet . . . but the fact is that our bodies appreciate and respond to regular food. I am not talking about five big meals a day – nor even five small meals – but breakfast, lunch, an evening meal and two small snacks in between. These will keep you from feeling hungry and therefore keep you happy – which is what will make you stick to the plan. So don't skip meals: eat everything you are allowed. And if you are one of the many people who has spent the past 20 years doing all the wrong things to try to slim, you may find my programme strange at first and feel you won't lose weight while eating so much. But you will!

Instructions applicable to all 10 weeks

**Plan what you are going to eat at least a day in advance;
shop up to a week in advance if possible.**

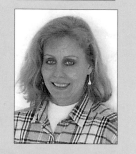
DAILY MILK ALLOWANCE

Every day on the plan you have an allowance of up to 200ml (⅓ pint) of skimmed milk. If you don't want this, have one 125ml (5fl oz) tub of low-fat natural Bio yoghurt instead – you need this for the calcium.

UNLIMITED

*Every day on the diet you can eat or drink any of the following
in addition to the meals, snacks and extras.*

Foods

- all fresh vegetables *(except potatoes and sweet potatoes, which should only be eaten as stated within the plans)*
- all fresh salad items. *In fact, you should eat as much fresh salad and lightly cooked or raw vegetables as possible, both at lunch time and in the evening.*

Cook without added fat: i.e., bake, steam, lightly boil, braise or microwave. Salads can be dressed with any of the 'unlimited' condiments above. Balsamic vinegar is excellent as it is so sweet and flavoursome, or use a dessertspoon of 70%-fat-free mayonnaise mixed with a little low-fat Bio yoghurt.

Drinks

- weak black tea or coffee (or with milk from allowance)
- fruit and herbal teas (unsweetened varieties)
- water
- mineral water
- Calorie-free drinks such as squashes, *mixers and fizzy drinks are best avoided as much as possible as they are full of additives, colorants and so on, and have little or no nutritional benefit.*

Condiments

- all fresh or dried herbs and spices
- a little salt (use sparingly)
- pepper
- lemon juice; lime juice
- chilli sauce
- mustard
- Worcestershire sauce
- light soy sauce
- vinegar
- sour pickles *(eg gherkins, onions)*
- oil-free French dressing
- tomato paste

FRUIT CHOICE

When 'fruit choice' is mentioned within the plans, choose one medium piece (e.g. an apple) or two small pieces (e.g. two plums) or one average portion (e.g. a medium plate of strawberries) of your choice. Bananas should be limited to one per day maximum and should be small. Eat as much citrus fruit as you can (within reason, very high quantities of citrus and some other fruits can cause problems). Be adventurous! Apples and bananas are marvellous food, but there is so much more out there waiting for you to try.

Always remember: fresh vegetables and salads are unlimited – eat as much of them as you can!

THE SIZEWISE FLYING START – WEEK 1 ONLY

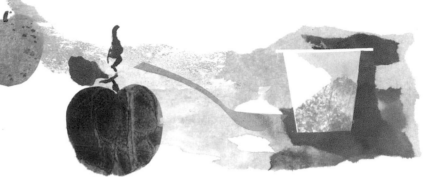

BREAKFAST

- Pick a Fruit Choice. Cut, segment or stir your fruit into a 125ml tub of low-fat natural Bio yoghurt or 100g pot of Diet Fruit Fromage Frais.
- Add a handful of Bran Flakes, Fruit'n Fibre, crushed Weetabix, Shredded Wheat or All Bran.
- Serve with 140ml (¼ pint) of orange juice.

MID-MORNING

- Choose one of the following:
  · 1 wholemeal crisp roll, plain or with yeast extract
  · 1 rye crispbread with yeast extract
  · 5 ready-to-eat dried apricots, peaches or prunes
  · 1 apple
  · crudités dipped in a little 70% fat-free mayonnaise mixed with low-fat Bio yoghurt.

LUNCH

either

Sandwich Lunch

- Using 2 slices of bread from a large medium-cut wholegrain loaf and a little low-fat spread, make a sandwich with one of the following fillings:
  · 100g (3½oz) tuna in brine
  · 1 hard-boiled egg
  · 50g (2oz) low-fat soft cheese
  · 50g (2oz) lean roast chicken
  · 40g (1½oz) Brie or Edam cheese
  · plus unlimited salad
  · *Follow with one fruit choice and I diet yoghurt (e.g. Shape).*

or

Salad Lunch

- Make a large salad and have it with one of the sandwich fillings above, plus I wholemeal bap or 50g (2oz) slice(s) of wholemeal French bread followed by one fruit choice and 1 yoghurt as above.

or

Hot Lunch

- Have one 225g (8oz) baked potato filled with one of the following:
  · 6 tablespoons baked beans
  · 50g (2oz) low-fat soft cheese (melt in microwave if liked)
  · 50g (2oz) canned tuna in brine, drained and mixed with 50g (2oz) butter beans and I dessertspoon 70% fat-free mayonnaise
- OR have 2 slices of bread as above, toasted and topped with one of the following:
  · 6 tablespoons baked beans
  · 1 poached egg
- plus one fruit choice and I diet yoghurt.

MID-AFTERNOON

- Fruit Choice

EVENING

- Choose one of these, plainly cooked *(all average sizes)*:
  · turkey steak
  · skinned chicken portion
  · white fish portion
  · small trout or salmon steak
  · 2 slices of lean roast meat
  · 1 vegetable burger
  · omelette of 2 size-3 eggs
- Add unlimited salad and/or vegetables, plus one medium (around 200g/7oz) portion of potato, pasta, rice or other grain, plainly cooked or 50g(2oz) bread.
- Add any of the following:
  · 1–2 tablespoons fat-free sauce or gravy
  · 1 level dessertspoon 70%-fat-free mayonnaise or relish

NOTE: *You could slice your protein/vegetables/salad and use your 'unlimited' condiments plus I level dessertspoon of honey to make a stir-fry, oiling the wok or pan with a little Fry Light cooking spray and adding a little fat-free stock as necessary.*

SizeWise Tips

Entertaining?

This is even better than eating out, as you are in control of what you prepare and serve. Choose from the recipes at the end of this workshop or scour the bookshops, slimming magazines and libraries for low-fat, low-cal recipes. Don't be afraid to try new ideas – apart from your make-up, hair and clothes, nothing dates you more than an outdated repertoire of recipes! As long as you don't want to entertain every other evening, you can still lose weight by following the plan extra carefully for the rest of the time.

Vegetarian?

That's fine – there are plenty of vegetarian choices within the meal selections. There are several vegetarian recipes, and others that can easily be adapted.

THE SIZEWISE EATING PLAN – WEEKS 2 TO 10

EXTRAS

EVERY DAY you may choose one or two of the following in addition to the rest of your diet, as explained in the instructions:

- I glass of dry or medium-dry wine
- 15g (½oz) butter or oil
- I frozen light chocolate mousse
- I tablespoon French dressing
- tablespoons half-fat cream
- tablespoons low-fat custard

SizeWise Tips

Eating out?

No-one expects you to live like a hermit while you lose weight. If eating out, you can control the number of calories you eat by choosing a main course and either a starter or a dessert, or by having fresh fruit for both starter and dessert (e.g. melon starter, fruit salad dessert); by declining the bread basket and butter; by avoiding main courses that are obviously high in fat, such as pastry dishes, anything coated and fried.

NOTE: Milk allowance, unlimiteds, fruit choices as week one.

INSTRUCTIONS Every day you will be eating a Breakfast, a Mid-morning Snack, a Lunch, a Mid-afternoon Snack, and an Evening Meal, plus either one or two items from a choice of Extras. *If you have a stone or less to lose:* Choose a SMALL BREAKFAST and pick just ONE Extra a day from the list. **If you have more than a stone to lose:** Choose a LARGE BREAKFAST and pick TWO Extras a day from the list. Now select your meals from the lists each day – and see the pounds melt away!

COLD BREAKFAST

small

- Same breakfast as Week One
- 40g (1½oz) muesli with milk from allowance; 1 fruit choice.
- 25g (1oz) unsweetened cereal of choice (e.g. Bran Flakes, Fruit'n Fibre) with milk from allowance; 1 large banana or 2 fruit choices.
- 25g (1oz) unsweetened cereal of choice with milk from allowance and 100g (3½ oz) fruit of choice chopped or mixed in plus 5 chopped dried apricots or prunes.
- 125ml tub of low-fat natural Bio yoghurt, with 1 teaspoon runny honey and 1 fruit choice.
- 1½ average slices of bread from a sliced loaf (preferably wholemeal), with a little low-fat spread and 2 teaspoons low-sugar jam or marmalade; 1 diet fruit yoghurt; 1 fruit choice.
- 25g (1oz) unsweetened cereal of choice with milk from allowance, 1 small slice of bread with a little low-fat spread and 1 teaspoon low-sugar jam or marmalade; ½ grapefruit or 1 kiwi fruit.

large

- Average (40g/1½oz) bowl of unsweetened cereal of choice (e.g. Branflakes, Fruit'n Fibre) with skimmed milk to cover (extra to allowance) and fruit choice (chopped in if liked); I slice of bread from a cut loaf (preferably wholemeal) with a little low-fat spread and 1 teaspoon low-sugar jam or marmalade or Marmite.
- 50g (2oz) no-added-sugar muesli with skimmed milk to cover (extra to allowance); 1 fruit choice.
- 2 slices of wholemeal bread from a large cut loaf with a little low-fat spread and 4 teaspoons low-sugar preserves; 1 large banana OR 1 fruit choice plus 1 diet yoghurt.
- Unlimited fresh fruit of choice or up to 50g/2oz ready-to-eat dried fruit chopped or mixed into 1 small tub of natural low-fat Bio yoghurt with 1 level teaspoon brown sugar or honey and 25g (1oz) unsweetened cereal of choice or 15g (½oz) muesli.

HOT BREAKFASTS

small

- 1 medium slice of toast with a little low-fat spread, topped with 1 small banana, sliced or mashed with a little lemon juice and cinnamon; 1 diet fruit yoghurt.
- 1 medium slice of toast spread with a little low-fat soft cheese and topped with 2 or 3 halved tomatoes, grilled, dry-fried in Fry Light spray or baked; 1 fruit choice.
- 1 medium egg, boiled or poached, with 1 medium slice toast and a little low-fat spread; 1 fruit choice.
- 1 average bowl of porridge, made with equal parts water and skimmed milk; 1 teaspoon brown sugar; 1 fruit choice.
- 1 medium slice of toast with a little low-fat spread, topped with 4 tablespoons baked beans; 1 citrus fruit.

large

- 1 medium egg, poached or fried in a pan coated with Fry Light spray; 4 tablespoons baked beans, 1 slice of extra-lean back bacon, grilled or dry-fried until crisp; 1 grilled tomato; 1 small slice of wholemeal bread with a little low-fat spread; ½ grapefruit.
- ½ can baked beans on 1 slice of toast from a large loaf; 1 fruit choice.
- Average bowlful of porridge made using half water and half skimmed milk with I level teaspoon sugar or honey; 1 slice of bread from a large medium-cut loaf with a little low-fat spread and Marmite; I fruit choice.
- Fruit compote and yoghurt – simmer one pack of mixed dried fruit in water to cover well until the fruit is tender and you have a rich fruity juice. Serve 5-6 pieces of the fruit and some of the juice with 150ml (¼ pint) low-fat natural Bio yoghurt; a handful of cereal flakes, preferably wholegrain, and 1 teaspoon runny honey. NB *By 'dried mixed fruit' I don't mean the mixed fruit for cake-making but the packs containing, usually, prunes, apricots, pear, peach and apple. Have 200 ml (⅓ pint) unsweetened orange juice with this breakfast.*

PACKED LUNCHES

• 2 medium slices of bread from a cut loaf (preferably wholemeal) with a little low-fat spread filled with plenty of fresh salad and one of the following:

· 1 hard-boiled egg and 1 teaspoon 70% fat-free mayonnaise (Kraft)
· 75g (3oz) peeled prawns and 1 teaspoon 70% fat-free mayonnaise
· 50g (2 packed slices) extra-lean ham and 1 teaspoon made mustard or pickle
· 50g (2oz) lean cooked chicken or turkey and 1 teaspoon 70% fat-free mayonnaise
· 25g (1oz) Edam or Brie or Philadelphia or Gouda or Jarlsberg or Danish Blue
· 40g (1½ oz) half-fat Cheddar or half-fat Edam or low-fat soft cheese or Feta
· 50g (2oz) smoked salmon, lemon juice and black pepper
· 25g (1oz) Parma ham and 4-5 cooked asparagus spears

PLUS (with any of above selections)
1 fruit choice and either 1 sachet low-calorie soup or 1 diet Shape yoghurt or diet Shape fromage frais.

• 1 large wholemeal bap with a little low-fat spread filled with plenty of fresh salad and one of the following:

· 25g (1oz) Cheddar and 1 teaspoon pickle
· 1 thin slice of extra-lean ham and 1 tablespoon cottage cheese
· 75g (3oz) lean cooked chicken (no skin)
· 50g (2oz) very lean roast beef and 1 teaspoon horseradish
· 50g (2oz) fresh poached salmon and 1 teaspoon mayonnaise
· ▪ 1 portion of Smoked Mackerel Pâté (page 31)

PLUS 1 large banana with any of the above.

• 1 pitta bread filled with plenty of fresh mixed salad and one of the following:

· 2 tablespoons hummus
· 1 tablespoon taramasalata
· 50g (2oz) Feta cheese, crumbled
· 100g (3½ oz) canned tuna in brine and 2-3 chopped stoned black olives
· 50g (2oz) reduced-fat liver pâté and chopped apple and orange

PLUS 2 fruit choices with any of the above.

• Flask of homemade Lentil and Vegetable Soup (*page 32*), with 1 average wholemeal roll; 1 diet yoghurt or fromage frais as above, 1 fruit choice

• 1 ready-made sandwich (from Boots or supermarkets, for instance) as long as it is calorie counted at 300 calories or less and contains plenty of salad (restrict to occasional use).

• 1 portion of homemade Mixed Bean and Pasta Salad (*page 33*), 1 large banana.

COLD LUNCHES AND SNACKS

• Any of the packed lunch ideas – have more salad on your plate than you would get in a sandwich.

• 1 portion of Fresh Tuna Salad (*page 33*) served with 1 small wholemeal roll with a little low-fat spread.

• Salad made by combining 50g (2oz) crumbled Feta cheese with one large chopped tomato, some chopped cucumber, crisp lettuce, 2 spring onions, 2 black olives, a little diced red pepper, in oil-free French dressing to taste; 1 mini pitta; 2 fruit choices or 1 banana.

• Low-fat Ploughman's: a 7.5cm (3in) slice of wholemeal French bread with a little low-fat spread; 40g (1½ oz) reduced-fat Cheddar cheese OR other reduced-fat hard cheese; large mixed salad with oil-free French dressing or a dash of balsamic vinegar; some celery sticks, 2 teaspoons sweet pickle; pickled onions.
NOTE *You can have 2 slices of extra lean ham or corned beef or 100g (3½ oz) tuna in brine or 75g (3oz) peeled prawns instead of the cheese).*

• Diet coleslaw with 1 slice of bread from a medium-cut loaf and a little low-fat spread, plus either 50g (2oz) lean cooked chicken or half-fat cheese or lean ham or vegetarian pâté.

• A chicken and fruit salad made by combining 75g (3oz) diced cooked chicken with 50g (2oz) each diced melon, orange and apple, all tossed in 2 tablespoons 70% fat-free mayonnaise mixed with 1 tablespoon skimmed milk and ½ teaspoon mild curry powder; 1 small wholemeal roll with low-fat spread; 1 diet fruit yoghurt.

• 1 portion Gazpacho Soup (*page 32*); 50g (2oz) wholegrain bread; 25g (1oz) Brie or Edam cheese.

• 1 portion Red Pepper Dip (*page 31*) with crudités, 50g (2oz) French bread, 1 large banana, 1 fruit choice.
NOTE *You can substitute 3 dark rye Ryvitas for any one slice of bread in the lunches.*

HOT LUNCHES AND SNACKS

• Any of the soup meals from packed lunches
• ½ can baked beans on 1 large slice of wholemeal toast; 1 large banana OR 2 scoops low-fat ice-cream (e.g. WeightWatchers); 1 satsuma or kiwi fruit or small portion of fresh berries.

• 300ml (½ pint) fresh vegetable, carrot or lentil soup from chilled counter, 1 wholemeal roll; 1 small slice of malt loaf or 1 crumpet with low-fat spread or 1 small tub of fruit yoghurt; 1 large banana or 2 fruit choices

• 250g (9oz) baked potato filled with 4 tablespoons baked beans or Chilli Chicken (*page 34*); lots of salad; 1 level tablespoon grated Parmesan cheese.

• 225g (8oz) baked potato filled with 4 tablespoons lentil dhal (canned) or with 2 tablespoons creamy dressing made by mixing together equal quantities of low-fat mayonnaise and low-fat Bio yoghurt with a dessertspoon low-fat crème fraîche (*optional*) and topped with 1 dessertspoon grated Parmesan cheese. Serve either with plenty of salad.

• 1 individual pizza base spread with 1 tablespoon pizza topping, covered with 4 thin slices of half-fat Mozzarella cheese OR 2 tablespoons half-fat ready-grated Mozzarella and finished with slices of tomato, mushroom and pepper; baked until bubbling and golden. Serve with plenty of salad.

• 1 cheese-and-tomato French bread pizza (frozen); lots of salad; 1 fruit choice.

• 2 medium eggs, scrambled with a little skimmed milk and seasoning (*no need to add butter to the pan*) on 2 medium slices of wholemeal bread with a little low-fat spread; 1 banana or 1 citrus fruit and 1 other fruit choice.

> **TIP**
> When selecting a banana for your fruit choice, for a change bake it in its own skin in a moderate oven for 20 minutes and serve hot with a little cream or custard from your day's Extra list.

MAIN MEALS

Red Meat and Poultry

- 1 medium pork steak, grilled, with 225g (8oz) new potatoes, 1 teaspoon butter, lots of vegetables and some apple sauce if liked.
- 110g (4oz) pork or lamb fillet, cubed and threaded on kebab stick with squares of red pepper and chunks of red onion; brushed with oil and grilled; served with 5 tablespoons boiled rice, 2 tablespoons heated Italian tomato sauce and lots of salad.

TIP: If you have time, marinate the meat first for a while in a little soy sauce or red wine.

- Average-sized chicken portion skinned and coated in a mixture of natural low-fat yoghurt and mild curry powder or tikka or tandoori powder (powder not paste); grilled or baked and served with 5 tablespoons plain boiled rice, 1 dessertspoon chutney and green salad.
- Average-sized chicken portion, grilled and skinned, and served with 200g (7oz) new potatoes, plenty of 'free' vegetables and either low-fat gravy or 2 tablespoons homemade Tomato Sauce *(page 35)*; 1 fruit choice.
- 1 small chicken breast portion, skinned, sliced and stir-fried with a selection of vegetables in 1 tablespoon groundnut or corn oil; seasonings of choice added, e.g. soy sauce, ginger, chilli, five-spice powder; 200g (7oz) (cooked weight) noodles or rice or pasta.
- Any ready-chilled or frozen meal for one labelled 'low in fat' and containing 400 calories or less (but don't choose this option more than once a week); large mixed salad or 2 or 3 vegetables; fruit choice.
- 110g (4oz) lean roast organic beef or 140g (5oz) lean roast chicken with small baked potato, several unlimited vegetables and 2 tablespoons wine gravy or skimmed pan juices and 1 teaspoon condiment of choice.

TIP: Toss a selection of root vegetables or Mediterranean vegetables in little olive oil and roast for 45 minutes, turning once. Count the oil as your day's Extra.

- 1 portion Chilli Chicken *(page 34)* with 6 tablespoons boiled basmati or fragrant rice or 1 chapati; large salad.
- 1 portion Chicken, Lime and Mango Brochettes *(page 35)* with 6 tablespoons boiled long-grain and wild rice; green salad.

Fish

- Any white fish fillet, cooked without added fat and served with potatoes boiled, mashed with skimmed milk or baked, plus peas, broccoli, carrots or other suitable vegetables and 1 dessertspoon sauce of choice.
- 1 small trout fried in Fry Light and served with 1 dessertspoon flaked toasted almonds, lemon juice, potatoes and vegetables.
- Monkfish or swordfish kebab: cube 200g (7oz) monkfish fillet and thread on kebab stick with tomato, 1 slice of lean bacon cut into squares, onion slices and courgette cubes. Brush with a little oil and grill. Serve with 2–3 tablespoons tomato sauce (e.g. Ragu or homemade, page 35) and 4 tablespoons plain boiled rice or noodles, and lots of salad.
- 1 salmon steak, topped with 1 tablespoon ready-made fresh pesto sauce and grilled on a baking sheet for 7–8 minutes; 200g (7oz) new potatoes, peas or broccoli.
- 1 portion of Spiced Salmon Fishcakes *(page 34)*; large mixed salad; 1 fruit choice.
- 1 portion of Whole Fish, Catalan-style *(page 34)*, 140g (5oz) new potatoes and large mixed salad.
- Salmon and broccoli risotto: Allow 50g (2oz) dry weight risotto rice per person; toss rice in non-stick frying pan with 15g (½ oz) butter to coat, add 140ml (5fl oz) well-flavoured vegetable or fish stock per person and simmer, stirring and adding more stock as you go. When rice is almost tender, add 75g (3oz) parboiled broccoli florets and 75g (3oz) flaked cooked salmon per person. Stir and serve with chopped parsley when rice is tender and still moist, seasoning to taste.

Pasta, Eggs and Vegetarian

- 50g (2oz) (raw weight) dried pasta of your choice, boiled and topped with either 5 tablespoons tomato sauce (e.g. Ragu or homemade) and 1 tablespoon grated Parmesan cheese (add sliced button mushrooms if you like) or topped with 2 tablespoons ready-made pesto sauce mixed with 1 large finely chopped fresh tomato and 1 small handful of pine nuts (optional) OR 100g (3½oz) any ready-made pasta sauce which doesn't contain cream. Serve with lots of salad.
- 2-egg omelette cooked in non-stick pan sprayed with Fry Light and filled with either sliced button mushrooms or a few prawns; served with 7.5cm (3 in) slice of French bread and salad OR 100g (3½oz) 5%-fat oven chips and salad.
- 50g (2oz) dry weight medium egg-thread noodles cooked according to packet instructions (usually boiled for up to 6 minutes) and tossed with a selection of thinly sliced vegetables stir-fried in 1 tablespoon groundnut or corn oil, soy sauce and 1 tablespoon black or yellow bean sauce. Add a little stock for a more moist stir-fry. Add 50g (2oz) lean sliced cooked chicken or turkey or pork or tofu or Quorn and stir-fry for a minute or two before serving.
- Any ready pasta, rice or vegetarian frozen or chilled meal labelled 'low fat' and containing 400 calories or less; large mixed salad or vegetables; fruit choice.

Limit convenience meals to one a week maximum.

- 1 Bird's-Eye Pizza for One, cheese and tomato only; large mixed salad.
- 1 Bird's-Eye Vegetable Quarter Pounder; 1 average wholemeal bap OR 200g (7oz) new potatoes; vegetables of choice or large salad; 1 dessertspoon relish of choice; 1 large banana.
- 1 portion Cantonese Vegetable Stir-fry *(see recipe, page 33)*; 50g (2oz) (dry weight) egg thread noodles or brown rice, boiled; 1 banana.
- 1 portion Goulash of Winter Vegetables and Beans *(see recipe, page 33)*; 40g (1½oz) (dry weight) brown rice, boiled.
- 1 portion Pasta with Pesto Tomato Sauce *(page 35)*; green salad.
- 1 portion Pasta Primavera *(page 35)*.

RECIPES

All recipes serve four, but most quantities can be halved to serve two. If cooking for one, some dishes can be frozen so you can cook for two or four and freeze the surplus. Such dishes are marked with an asterisk (✳).

AVOCADO LIME DIP

125 calories; 12g fat per serving;
good source of
vitamin E

- *2 well-ripened medium avocados*
- *juice of 1 good lime*
- *few drops of Tabasco sauce*
- *little salt*
- *black pepper*
- *chopped coriander leaves, to garnish (optional)*

Peel and stone the avocados and mash the flesh in a small bowl. Add the lime juice, Tabasco and seasoning and combine well.

Serve garnished with the coriander leaves if you like.

The dip can also be used as a crispbread or open sandwich topping, and will keep in an airtight jar in the fridge for a few days if covered completely with a thin film of olive oil. Pour the oil off before serving.

SMOKED MACKEREL PÂTÉ ✳

130 calories; 9g fat per serving
good source of
omega-3 oils, protein,
calcium, vitamin B[3]

- *175g (6oz) smoked mackerel fillet*
- *100g (3½ oz) 8%-fat fromage frais*
- *2 tablespoons natural low-fat Bio yoghurt*
- *juice of ½ lemon*
- *1 good teaspoon horseradish sauce*
- *little salt*
- *black pepper*
- *chopped parsley or dill, to garnish*

Put all the ingredients except the garnish in a blender and blend to a smooth paste. Adjust the seasoning, chill and serve garnished with the parsley or dill.

RED PEPPER DIP

65 calories; 2g fat per serving
good source of:
beta-carotene, vitamin C, fibre

- *2 large red peppers*
- *100g (3½ oz) 8%-fat fromage frais*
- *few drops of Tabasco sauce*
- *little salt*
- *black pepper*
- *paprika, to garnish*

Halve and deseed the peppers and place on a baking sheet, skin sides up. Cook under hot grill until the skins have bubbled and blackened, then remove from heat and place in a plastic bag. Leave for 5 minutes, when the skins will come off easily (leave a few black bits of skin on the peppers to add a barbecue-type flavour to the dip).

Chop peppers coarsely and place in blender with remaining ingredients apart from the garnish. Blend to a smooth dip consistency.

Chill and serve garnished with paprika.

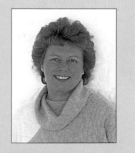

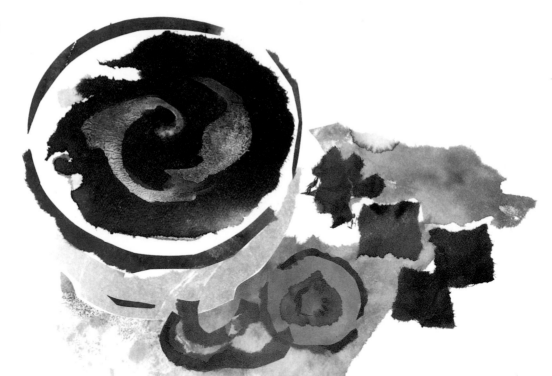

LENTIL AND VEGETABLE SOUP *

200 calories; 5g fat per serving

good source of
fibre, magnesium, iron, vitamin E,
B vitamins, vitamin C

- 1 tablespoon sunflower oil
- 1 large onion, finely chopped
- 1-2 teaspoons curry powder (optional)
- 1 litre (2 pints) fat-free vegetable or chicken stock
- 110g (4oz) uncooked brown or green lentils
- 1 large leek, cleaned and chopped
- 1 large parsnip, peeled and chopped
- 2 medium carrots, chopped
- 100g (3½oz) swede or sweet potato
- 100g (3½oz) butternut squash
- 200g (7oz) potato, peeled and chopped
- 2 celery stalks, chopped
- 1 good dessertspoon tomato paste
- 1 teaspoon sun-dried tomato purée (optional)
- little salt
- black pepper

Heat the oil in a large saucepan and sauté the onion until soft. Add the curry powder, if using, and stir for a minute or two. Add the stock and lentils and simmer for 45 minutes or until lentils are tender

Add the remaining ingredients and simmer for another 45 minutes.

Transfer half the soup to a blender and blend until smooth. Return the blended soup to the saucepan, heat through and serve.

WATERCRESS AND PEA SOUP *

112 calories; 4g fat per serving

good source of
vitamin C, beta-carotene, fibre, iron

- 15g (½oz) butter
- 1 medium mild onion or 4-5 shallots, peeled and chopped
- 825ml (1½ pints) vegetable or chicken stock
- 325g (12oz) petits pois or tender frozen peas
- 1 large pack or 2 bunches of watercress, picked over and large stalks removed
- little salt
- black pepper
- 1 tablespoon chopped mint

Melt the butter in a saucepan and sauté the onion or shallots until soft. Add the stock, peas and watercress and simmer for 10-15 minutes.

Season, then put the soup in a blender and blend until almost smooth (only a few seconds). Return the soup to the pan and reheat, stirring the mint in for the last minute.

Variations: *you can cook the same recipe using fresh parsley instead of watercress. You can also add some boiled floury potato to either of these recipes for a thicker, more substantial soup. 2 chunks of potato added would add about 25 calories and no fat per portion.*

GAZPACHO SOUP

120 calories; 4g fat per serving

good source of
beta-carotene, vitamin C, fibre

- 1 large green pepper, deseeded and chopped into small cubes
- 450g (1lb) cucumber, peeled and chopped
- 1 mild Spanish onion, peeled and finely chopped
- 1 garlic clove, peeled and chopped
- 1 large can (400g/14oz) peeled plum tomatoes OR 6 large ripe tomatoes, skinned, deseeded and chopped, including juice
- 1 tablespoon red wine vinegar
- 1 tablespoon olive oil
- 3 tablespoons tomato paste
- pinch of chilli powder or dash of Tabasco sauce
- 2 tablespoons freshly chopped parsley
- 2 medium slices of brown bread

Reserve 1 tablespoon each of the pepper, cucumber and onion. Blend the rest of the ingredients, except the parsley and bread, in a blender and dilute to a thickish soup with water. Stir well and chill for an hour or two in the fridge.

Make croutons by cutting the bread into 1cm (½in) squares and baking in a medium hot oven for 10 minutes or until golden and crisp.

Serve the chilled soup garnished with a little of the reserved pepper, cucumber, onion, parsley and croutons each.

MIXED BEAN AND PASTA SALAD

265 calories; 5g fat per serving

good source of
fibre, protein, vitamin C

- 150g (5½oz) (dry weight) pasta shells, boiled and drained
- 100g (3½oz) broad beans, cooked
- 400g (14 oz) canned mixed beans, drained
- 1 beef tomato, deseeded and chopped
- 4 spring onions, chopped
- 2 tablespoons freshly chopped parsley
- 5 tablespoons oil-free French dressing
- 1 tablespoon olive oil
- pinch of caster sugar

Combine all the dry ingredients in a bowl. In another small bowl, combine the oil-free French dressing with the olive oil and sugar. Pour this dressing over the salad, stir gently and serve.

NUTTY RICE SALAD

350 calories; 8g fat per serving

good source of
B vitamins, vitamin E, fibre, protein

- 200g (7oz) (raw weight) brown rice, boiled and cooled slightly
- 4 rings of fresh pineapple (or canned in juice), chopped
- 1 red apple, cored and chopped (including skin)
- 1 tablespoon pine nuts
- 2 tablespoons toasted flaked almonds
- 1 large banana, peeled and sliced
- 200g (7oz) cooked chicken, skin removed and diced OR 200g (7oz) tofu chunks
- 8 tablespoons oil-free French dressing
- 1 tablespoon fresh chopped coriander leaves (optional)

Combine all the ingredients except the coriander. Serve immediately, garnished with the coriander.

FRESH TUNA SALAD

260 calories; 6.5g fat per serving

good source of
fibre, vitamin E, omega-3 oils, vitamin C, B-group vitamins, calcium, protein, iron

- little Fry Light olive oil cooking spray
- 400g (14 oz) fresh tuna steak, cut into chunks
- 4 Little Gem lettuce heads OR 2 butter-head lettuces
- 400g (14oz) canned cannellini beans, drained
- I yellow pepper, deseeded and sliced
- 8 black olives, stoned and halved
- 1 small red onion, thinly sliced
- 12 cherry tomatoes
- 2 hard-boiled eggs, shelled and quartered
- 4 tablespoons oil-free French dressing

Spray a non-stick frying pan with the Fry Light and heat. When hot, add the tuna chunks and sear the outsides until golden. Turn the heat down and continue cooking for a minute or two until the fish is just tender. Leave to cool slightly.

Meanwhile quarter the lettuces, removing any discoloured outer leaves and arrange on a serving platter. Add the beans, tuna, pepper, olives, onion, tomatoes and eggs in separate small piles on the platter between the lettuce quarters.

Spoon the dressing over to serve.

Note: *good-quality canned tuna can be used, in which case there is no need to fry it.*

CANTONESE VEGETABLE STIR-FRY

126 calories; 6g fat per serving

good source of
fibre, protein, vitamin C, vitamin E, beta-carotene

- 1 tablespoon sesame oil
- 200g (7oz) tofu or Quorn chunks
- 50g (2oz) baby sweetcorn
- 100g (3½oz) mange-tout peas
- 150g (5½oz) carrots, cut into strips or ribbons
- 150g (5½oz) broccoli, cut into small florets
- 100g (3½oz) Chinese leaves
- 100g (3½oz) fresh beansprouts
- 4 spring onions
- 1 small knob of ginger, chopped
- 1 teaspoon Chinese five-spice powder
- 2 tablespoons light soy sauce
- 125 ml (4½fl oz) vegetable stock
- 1 teaspoon cornflour

Heat the oil in a wok or large frying pan and stir-fry the tofu or Quorn to colour. Add the sweetcorn, mange-tout peas, carrot and broccoli and stir-fry for 3 minutes. Add the Chinese leaves, beansprouts, spring onions, ginger and five-spice powder and stir-fry again for 2 minutes, adding a little soy sauce and a little vegetable stock towards the end of this time.

Combine the remaining vegetable stock with the cornflour and remaining soy sauce and add to the pan, stirring until the sauce thickens.

GOULASH OF WINTER VEGETABLES AND BEANS *

230 calories; 6g fat per serving

good source of
fibre, beta-carotene, vitamin C

- 1 tablespoon sunflower oil
- 2 medium onions, peeled and sliced
- 3 medium carrots, peeled and chopped
- 4 celery stalks, chopped
- 1 level tablespoon Hungarian paprika
- 225g (8oz) potatoes, cut into small chunks
- 1 parsnip, cubed
- 200g (7oz) orange-fleshed squash OR 100g (3½oz) sweet potato
- 400g (14oz) canned tomatoes
- 150g (5½oz) cooked red kidney beans
- 1 tablespoon tomato paste
- 2 teaspoons mixed herbs
- 400ml (14fl oz) vegetable stock
- little salt
- black pepper
- 3 tablespoons half-fat crème fraîche

Heat oil in a flameproof casserole and soften the onion in it for a few minutes. Stir in carrot and celery. Cook for 5 minutes.

Add the paprika, stir for a minute then add the rest of the ingredients, except the crème fraîche and stir well. Simmer for 1 hour, or until everything is tender and you have a rich sauce.

Adjust the seasoning and add the crème fraîche to serve.

(* Undercook slightly before freezing)

SPICED SALMON FISHCAKES WITH A CREAMED CAPER SAUCE *

280 calories; 13g fat per serving

good source of
omega-3 oils, vitamin E,
vitamin B6, protein

- 350g (12½oz) salmon fillet, lightly poached, microwaved or baked and flaked
- 350g (12½oz) old potatoes, boiled until just tender and roughly mashed with pinch of hot paprika or dash of Tabasco sauce
- 1 teaspoon chopped fresh or freeze-dried lemon grass
- juice of 1 small lime
- 1 tablespoon chopped coriander leaves
- pinch of ground ginger
- 1 small red pepper, deseeded, finely chopped and blanched or microwaved for 1 minute
- little salt
- black pepper
- 2 small eggs, beaten

for the sauce:
- 4 tablespoons low-fat natural Bio yoghurt
- 1 tablespoon half-fat crème fraîche
- 1 level tablespoon chopped well-drained capers

In a bowl, combine all the fishcake ingredients except the egg with a fork, making sure to leave at least some visible pieces of salmon. Now add the beaten egg, mixing gently.

Form the mixture into 8 small patties (they will be pretty soft but don't worry) and place on a lightly oiled baking sheet. Either bake for 20 minutes in a preheated medium hot oven or grill under a medium heat for 10 minutes, turning once, or until cakes are lightly golden.

Meanwhile, combine the sauce ingredients. When the fishcakes are cooked, serve with the sauce.

* Fishcakes will freeze; sauce won't.

WHOLE FISH, CATALAN STYLE *

250 calories; 9g fat per serving

good source of
calcium, protein,
beta-carotene, vitamin C

- 1 tablespoon olive oil
- 1 large Spanish onion, finely chopped
- 1 large green pepper, deseeded and coarsely chopped
- 2 garlic cloves, crushed
- 400g (14oz) canned chopped tomatoes
- 4 tablespoons passata
- 1 tablespoon tomato paste
- pinch of brown sugar
- 16 black olives, stoned
- 1 teaspoon each fresh rosemary, basil, thyme
- little salt
- black pepper
- 4 tilapia fish or red mullet, ready-cleaned and scaled

Heat the oil in a large saucepan or small frying pan and sauté the onion and green pepper until soft and just turning golden. Add the garlic and cook for a minute or two. Add the rest of the ingredients except the fish, bring to simmer and cook for 30 minutes or until you have a rich sauce.

About 15 minutes from the end of cooking time, grill the fish under a moderate to high heat for 8–10 minutes.

Serve the fish with the sauce.

Note: *this sauce recipe makes a good basic tomato sauce if you omit the green pepper and olives.*

* Sauce only.

CHILLI CHICKEN *

255 calories; 13g fat per serving

good source of
protein, vitamins C and E, beta-carotene

- 1 tablespoon sunflower or corn oil
- 1 medium red onion, sliced
- 450g (1lb) skinless, boneless chicken, cut into strips
- 1 large red pepper, deseeded and sliced
- 2 teaspoons Jerk or Cajun seasoning (more or less to taste)
- 1 courgette, thinly sliced
- 2 rings of fresh pineapple (or canned in juice)
- 1 small ripe avocado, peeled, stoned and chopped (do this just before you are ready to cook or the avocado will discolour)

Heat the oil in a large non-stick frying pan or wok and stir-fry the onion and chicken over a medium to high heat until the chicken is golden and the onion partly cooked, about 3 minutes.

Turn the heat down slightly, add the pepper and Jerk or Cajun seasoning and stir-fry for 2–3 minutes, until you can catch the aromas coming from the pan. Add the courgette and pineapple and stir-fry for another minute. Add the avocado, stir and serve.

Variation: *for a milder dish, add a little all-spice instead of the Jerk or Cajun seasoning.*

* Freeze without the avocado. Add avocado when reheating.

CHICKEN, LIME AND MANGO BROCHETTES WITH A MINT RAITA SAUCE *

230 calories; 9g fat per serving
good source of
protein, magnesium, B vitamins, beta-
carotene, vitamin C

- *3 limes*
- *1 garlic clove, finely chopped*
- *2 cm (¾in) piece of fresh ginger, finely chopped*
- *2 tablespoons sunflower or groundnut oil*
- *1 good dessertspoon runny honey*
- *2 tablespoons light soy sauce*
- *little salt*
- *black pepper*
- *4 boneless chicken breasts, each weighing about 125g (4½ oz), skinned and cubed*
- *1 ripe mango*

for the mint raita:
- *4 tablespoons half-fat Greek-style yoghurt*
- *1 tablespoon chopped fresh mint*

Several hours before you plan to eat, begin to marinate the chicken. Grate the rind off one of the limes and reserve it. Juice 2 of the limes and add the juice to a glass or ceramic dish. Add the rind, garlic, ginger, oil, honey, soy sauce, salt and seasoning to the dish and combine well with a wooden spoon. Add the chicken pieces and toss them well in the marinade. Cover and leave to marinate for up to 12 hours.

When ready to cook, peel and cube the mango and thread it with the chicken on skewers. Grill under a medium heat, turning once, for about 8 minutes, basting with any remaining sauce once or twice.

Meanwhile, make the sauce: combine the yoghurt with the mint.

When the brochettes are cooked, serve them with any pan juices, the remaining lime cut into quarters, and the raita.

* Brochettes can be frozen cooked or uncooked. Sauce will not freeze.

PASTA WITH PESTO TOMATO SAUCE *

425 calories; 22g fat per serving
good source of
calcium, vitamin C, vitamin E and beta-carotene

- *2 good garlic cloves, peeled*
- *1 pack or pot of fresh basil, stalks removed*
- *little salt*
- *2 tablespoons pine nuts*
- *50g (2oz) fresh grated Parmesan cheese*
- *4 medium-ripe large tomatoes, skinned, deseeded and finely chopped*
- *4 tablespoons olive oil*
- *275g (10oz) pappardelle pasta (dry weight)*

Using a pestle and mortar, pound the garlic with the basil and salt until you have a rough purée. Add the pine nuts and pound again, then add the cheese and mix that well in. If there is enough room in your mortar, add the tomatoes and pound again for a minute or two (otherwise transfer to a strong mixing bowl and beat thoroughly with a wooden spoon). Lastly pour in the oil and mix to combine.

Cook the pasta until al dente in plenty of lightly salted boiling water, about 10 minutes. Serve the sauce poured over the piping-hot drained pasta.

* You can freeze the sauce fairly successfully, or it will keep in an airtight container for a week or more in the fridge.

PASTA PRIMAVERA

450 calories; 9.5g fat per serving
good source of
fibre, vitamin C,
calcium, beta-carotene

- *300g (11oz) pasta spirals or penne (dry weight)*
- *150g (5½oz) baby broad beans*
- *4 small courgettes, sliced*
- *200g (7oz) baby carrots*
- *1 tablespoon olive oil*
- *8 tender asparagus tips*
- *50g (2oz) fresh baby peas*
- *4 baby leeks, halved lengthwise and each half cut into two*
- *8 spring onions*
- *100ml (3½oz) low-fat crème fraîche*
- *50g (2oz) 8%-fat fromage frais*
- *50ml (2 fl oz) skimmed milk*
- *50g (2oz) fresh grated Parmesan cheese*
- *2 teaspoons French mustard*
- *little salt*
- *black pepper*
- *2 tablespoons chopped fresh parsley, to garnish*

Put a pan of lightly salted water on to boil for the pasta.

Parboil the broad beans, courgettes and carrots in lightly salted water for 2 minutes and drain thoroughly.

Meanwhile, put the pasta in the boiling pasta water. Heat the olive oil in a non-stick frying pan.

Put the asparagus, peas and leeks in a steamer set over a saucepan of boiling water. Steam for a few minutes until just cooked.

While the pasta is boiling and the vegetables are steaming, fry the broad beans, courgettes, carrots and spring onions in the olive oil over a medium heat until slightly golden, but still with some bite (a few minutes), stirring once or twice.

Combine the crème fraîche, fromage frais, skimmed milk, cheese, mustard and seasoning in a small bowl. When the pasta is cooked, about 10 minutes, drain and toss with the steamed vegetables, the fried vegetables and the crème fraîche sauce.

Garnish with the parsley to serve.

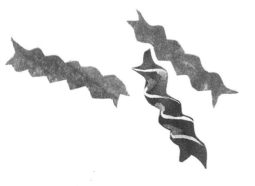

This simple tone, strength and stretch programme devised and demonstrated by top UK personal trainer, Louise Taylor, RSA, will work fast to help you recover a more youthful shape and body definition. It lets you work hardest on the areas of your body that are most in need of attention.

NOTE If you have arthritis or any medical condition which you think may prevent you from exercising or if you have done no exercise at all recently, check with your doctor first (see Rejuvenating Joints, page 51).

WORKSHOP 3 SHAPEWISE 1 – TOTAL TONE

Before You Begin

Please do read these notes and follow all the advice carefully every time you exercise. Bodies that haven't been used to exercise in some time need nurturing, not punishing – it is very important always to exercise within your own capabilities.

The basic TOTAL TONE programme consists of a three-minute **WARM-UP**, followed by five short **WARM-UP STRETCHES**, then 10 minutes of nine key **TOTAL TONE EXERCISES**, followed by two to three minutes of **COOL-DOWN STRETCHES**, which will also help your flexibility and posture.

This will give you a 20-minute programme in all, which you will be doing three times a week *(see the schedules beginning on page 8).* **Don't exercise immediately after eating, or when ill or very tired. A stamina – building aerobic programme is detailed in Workshop 14.**

Don't skip any of the moves, particularly the warm-up and stretches – if you don't warm up and cool down properly you'll find the Total Tone exercises harder to do, and you will be more inclined to suffer muscular ache.

• Run through the moves slowly at first and pay close attention to Louise's posture throughout – it's better to do an exercise once well, than eight repeats ('reps') incorrectly. Having said that, you can't expect an under-used body to cope with all the moves perfectly at first – e.g., you may not be able to achieve the same degree of stretch that Louise achieves in the photos at first, or be able to hold an identical 'finish' position in all of the exercises. Don't worry! You will see and feel improvement week by week – as long as you keep trying your very best.

• After the basic Total Tone programme described above, there are four short optional add-on sections if you want to do EXTRA work on your main problem areas. Simply add on whichever extra section(s) you want to do (using the shape assessment results you found on page 21 for help, if necessary) and then add it on to your session AFTER the basic Total Tone Exercises and BEFORE the cool-down stretches. However, don't attempt this extra work until you have been doing the basic programme for at least two weeks and can do it well.

• The Total Tone programme is to be done three times a week (four, if you like, later) with rest days in between. So don't do your three sessions three days in a row – space them out evenly during the week. Your body needs a chance to recover and adapt.

• Wear suitable comfortable clothing, e.g. t-shirt or leotard and leggings or shorts. Until you are thoroughly warmed up, wear extra layers (e.g. a tracksuit) and use these to keep warm during the cool-down. Cold muscles are susceptible to injury. Wear proper training shoes.

TIME TO WARM UP . . .

Take three minutes to warm up all your major muscles. Take deep even breaths throughout, and work up to a good momentum, with a smooth rhythm.

1 First do some marching on the spot. Tummy tucked in, head high, shoulders back but relaxed and down; march with arms swinging gently, gradually marching a little higher and arms pumping a little harder. March for about 30 seconds.

2 Now move on to 'step touches' take a fairly big step to the right with your right foot, then bring left foot to meet it. Take a step to the left and bring right foot to meet left. As you do so, begin circling your arms – first small circles, then larger ones. Step-touch for 30 seconds. Now carry on step-touching, but this time punch your arms (fists closed) up towards ceiling and back down. Reach! Step-touch and reach for 30 seconds.

3 Next, do double step-touches – take one pace to the right side, bring left foot to join right, then take one more pace to the right. Repeat to the left side. Move lightly across the floor, making the middle step into a small hop. As you go, lift your arms out straight to sides and up, then bring them back down again. Do double step-touches for 30 seconds. By now you should be feeling quite warm.

4 Do 30 seconds of hamstring curls. With feet hip-width apart, bring right heel up behind you, bending right knee. Feel back of your right thigh working. Return to the floor and curl with other leg. Keep curling alternately and as you do each curl, swing your arms up in front of you.

5 Finish with half a minute of 'toe taps'. With legs just over hip-width apart and weight on left leg, point and tap right toe out to side; lightly transfer weight on to right leg and repeat with left toe. Repeat these taps and, as you do so, lift arms alternately to reach overhead. Now you are warm. (If you aren't, do the warm up again, putting plenty of effort into it.)

WARM-UP STRETCHES
Hold each for a count of 8 and breathe normally.

1 INNER THIGH AND SIDE STRETCH
Stand with legs wide apart, tummy tucked in. With right foot turned out, bend right knee and, keeping left leg straight, bend over to the right, stretching left arm out as shown and with right forearm resting lightly on right thigh to support the spine. Repeat to the other side.

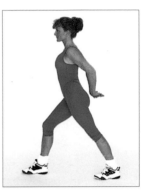

2 CALF AND CHEST STRETCH
Stand as shown, tummy tucked in, with left leg back and right knee bent, keeping body weight slightly forward. Clasp hands behind back and push the chest forward. Feel the stretch in your right calf and across your chest. Repeat with the other leg.

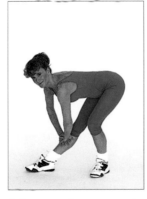

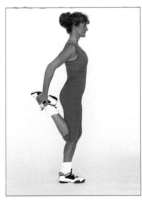

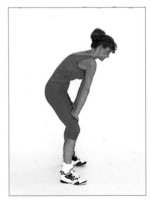

3 HAMSTRING (BACK OF THIGH) STRETCH
Stand as shown, with left leg behind right and left knee bent. Keeping right leg straight, bend over right leg and lift buttocks high, placing hands below right knee for support, until you feel a stretch in your right hamstring. Repeat to other side.

4 STANDING QUADRICEPS (FRONT THIGH) STRETCH
Stand, tummy tucked in, feet hip-width apart, well balanced. Raise right foot behind you as shown and clasp foot behind you, using right hand. Bring heel in to touch bottom. Slowly release and repeat to the other side.

5 BACK STRETCH
Stand with feet hip-width apart, tummy tucked in and hands resting halfway down thighs. Now curl your back into a letter 'c', pulling tummy in towards your spine as you do, then relax. Repeat four times in a slow and controlled manner.
That finishes your warm up.

THE TOTAL TONE EXERCISES

A Note About Repetitions

Build up over a few sessions to repeating each exercise for the stated number of reps. If you are unused to exercise, you may find you can only do a few reps to begin with, but you will soon get stronger. Work to the point where the muscle being worked tells you it has done enough (a slight trembling in the muscle is a good indication), do one more, then stop and move on to the next exercise. Stop for a few seconds after each block of eight reps, if you like. Breathe normally throughout unless instructed otherwise. Once you have done the programme several times at the full amount of reps, you can do more to keep progress going, again stopping when your working muscle tells you it has done enough.

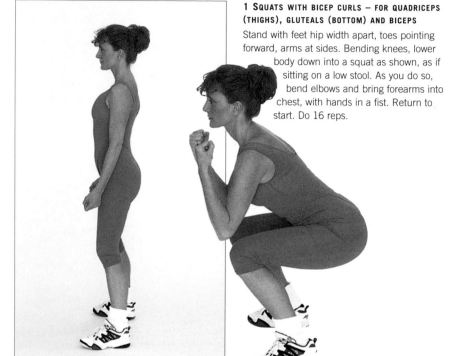

1 SQUATS WITH BICEP CURLS – FOR QUADRICEPS (THIGHS), GLUTEALS (BOTTOM) AND BICEPS

Stand with feet hip width apart, toes pointing forward, arms at sides. Bending knees, lower body down into a squat as shown, as if sitting on a low stool. As you do so, bend elbows and bring forearms into chest, with hands in a fist. Return to start. Do 16 reps.

2 PLIÉS WITH TRICEPS EXTENSIONS – FOR INNER THIGH AND TRICEPS (BACK OF UPPER ARMS)

Stand with legs wide apart, toes pointing outwards, arms at sides as shown. Keeping feet flat on the floor, chest up and tummy tucked in, bend at the knees and lower your body until your thighs are parallel to the floor (or as low as you can get if not that low). As you do so, bring your arms straight out behind you as shown, keeping shoulders relaxed and palms facing inwards. Return to start and do 16 reps.

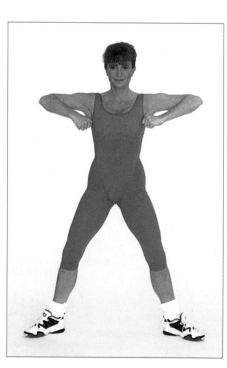

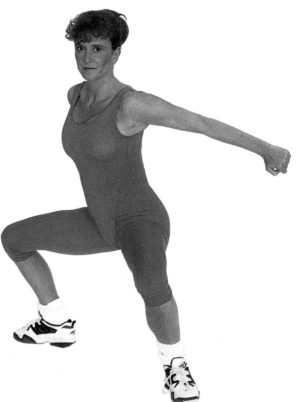

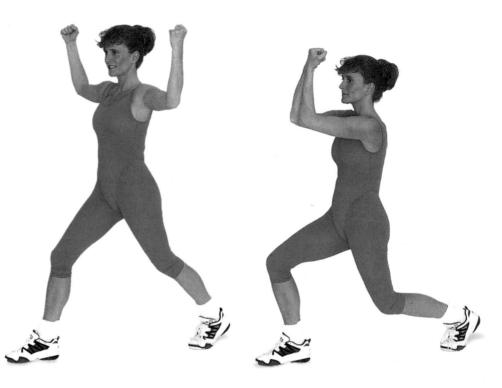

3 FORWARD LUNGES WITH PECTORAL FLIES – FOR QUADRICEPS, HAMSTRING, GLUTEALS PECTORALS (CHEST)

Stand with feet hip-width apart and arms raised at your sides as shown. Take a big step forward on your right leg, bending both knees to 90°. Keep your right knee over your heel and lift left heel off floor. As you do, bring elbows and forearms to meet in front of your chest. Return to starting position for arms and legs, repeat with left leg and arms. Do 8 reps on each leg, alternately.

4 ABDOMINAL CRUNCHES – FOR ABDOMINALS (STOMACH)

Now lie on your back on your mat or towel, fingers lightly placed behind head, knees bent as shown, feet flat on floor and tummy pulled in towards the floor. Now, breathing out, lift your head and tops of shoulders off the floor, using your stomach muscles to bring you up, NOT your hands or neck. Keep your chin off your chest. Make the movement controlled. Slowly lower. Repeat 16 times. If your neck begins to ache, stop – this means your stomach muscles are tired.

EXERCISE PROFILE

Sue

By the end of week four, Sue has got 2 inches off her hips and 1½ inches off her waist and is really enjoying her exercise. Her stamina is already excellent and, she says, 'I feel better and more full of energy.'

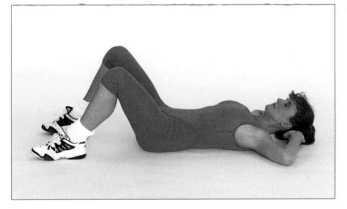

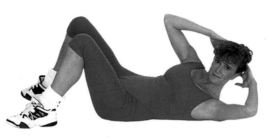

5 DIAGONAL CRUNCHES – FOR WAIST

In the same starting position as previous exercise, come up again, but this time bring your right arm and shoulder across towards your left knee, slowly lower, then bring your left shoulder up towards your right knee. Lower and do 16 reps each side, alternately.

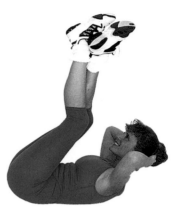

6 DOUBLE CRUNCHES – FOR ABDOMINALS

Same starting position as previous two exercises. Now raise legs in air as shown, with ankles crossed and knees slightly bent. Come up as in the abdominal crunches, but this time try to lift your buttocks off the floor at the same time as you raise your shoulders. Pause, then release to the floor. Breathe out as you lift and keep chin lifted; inhale as you lower. Do 8 reps.

7 SIDE LEG RAISES – FOR HIPS AND OUTER THIGHS

Turn on to your right side and lie as shown, with your right leg bent, left leg straight but knee relaxed. Keeping hips stacked (don't allow left hip to slip back, or the exercise will be less effective), slowly lift left leg (not too high), leading with your heel. Lower slowly. Keep buttocks tightly clenched throughout. Do 32 reps, then turn over and do 32 on the other side.

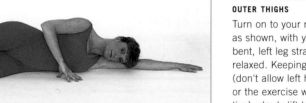

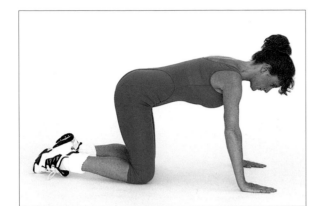

8 PRESS-UPS — FOR PECTORALS AND TRICEPS (BACK OF UPPER ARMS)

Kneel on all fours, keeping your back straight and tummy tucked in, fingers pointing forwards. Now slowly lower your body so that your forehead nearly touches the floor. (Don't dip your head to do this; keep it aligned with your back.) Return to start position. Do 12 reps.

9 BACK EXTENSIONS — FOR LOWER BACK

Lie face down on floor, resting your head on your hands as shown. Now lIft your upper body and arms a few inches off the floor. (Don't use your feet as a pivot while doing this; use your back muscles.) Always look at the floor. Slowly return to start. Repeat 12 times.

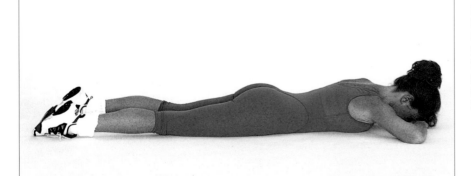

COOL-DOWN STRETCHES

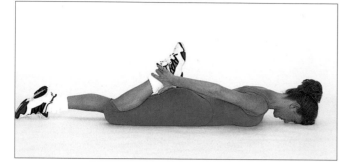

1 QUADRICEPS STRETCH

Lie on your front, arms at sides. Bend your right knee and bring your right foot in towards your bottom. Hold your right foot with your right hand and gently pull your foot a little further down, to feel a good stretch along the front of your right thigh. Hold for a count of 8, relax and repeat to other side.

2 CALF STRETCH

Turn over and lie on your back, knees bent, feet on floor. Lift your right leg into the air as shown and flex your foot as hard as you can, trying to get your toes pointing as far down towards your head as possible. Feel a stretch along your right calf. Hold for a count of 12. Bring leg down to start and repeat the stretch with left leg.

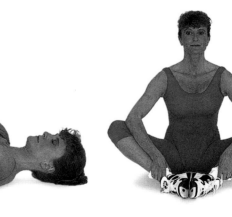

3 HAMSTRING STRETCH

Lying in the same start position as for calf stretch, bring your right leg in towards your chest, clasping your hand behind your thigh as shown and straightening out your leg as much as possible. Feel the stretch all along the back of your right thigh. Hold for a count of 16, trying to straighten out the leg a little more towards the end of the stretch. Return to start and repeat with the other leg.

4 LOWER BACK STRETCH

From the same start position as for calf stretch, slowly bring knees in to your chest, using your hands to pull them in a little further as you do. Feel a stretch in your lower back. Hold for a count of 12.

5 INNER THIGH STRETCH

Now sit up and place the soles of your feet together in front of you. Keeping lower back strong (don't slump), place hands on ankles as shown and gently push each thigh down towards the floor with your elbows until you feel a stretch along each inner thigh. Hold for a count of 12.

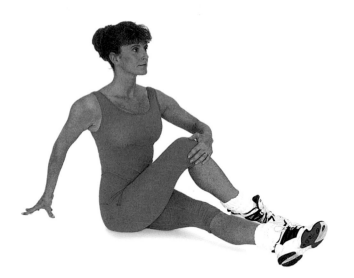

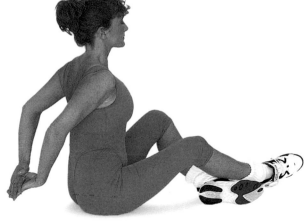

6 GLUTEAL STRETCH

Still sitting, with left leg straight on the floor, bring right foot over left leg and place it on the floor near your left knee. With left hand, gently press the knee towards your chest. Feel the stretch in right buttock muscle. Hold for a count of 8. Repeat to other side.

7 CHEST STRETCH

Still sitting, with your legs in a comfortable position in front of you, clasp hands behind your back, palms facing outwards, and pull your arms out away from your body. Feel a stretch across your chest. Hold for a count of 8.

10 SIDE STRETCH

Still sitting, place right hand on the floor and bring left arm up towards the ceiling and over your head; leaning over to the right slightly as you do so. Feel a stretch all along your left side. Hold for a count of 8 and repeat to the other side.

That completes your basic Total Tone Exercises. Don't forget to add on any of the following exercises for your particular 'trouble spots' if you like – they should be done BEFORE the cool down.

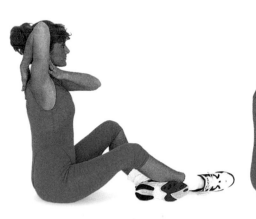

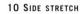

8 TRICEP STRETCH

Sitting in the same position as previous stretch, raise your right arm above your head and bend your elbow, putting hand, palm inwards, in the centre of your upper back. Using your left hand press your right arm backwards to feel a stretch along your tricep (back of upper arm). Hold for a count of 8. Return to start and repeat with left arm.

9 UPPER BACK STRETCH

Still in the same sitting position, bring your arms out in front of you and clasp fingers, palms outwards. Now push your hands away from your body until you feel a stretch across your upper back. Hold for a count of 8.

ADD-ONS... ADD-ONS... ADD-ONS...

Waist and Stomach

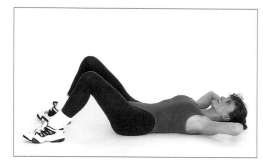

PULSING CRUNCHES

Lie on your back with knees bent, feet flat on floor, fingers loosely clasped behind head, elbows wide. Pull stomach in towards floor and, using abdominal muscles, lift head and upper back off floor as shown. Instead of returning to the floor as in the basic crunches on page 39, return just halfway to floor before coming up again, and repeat 16 times. Make these pulsing movements faster than ordinary crunches. *And remember — your head doesn't touch the floor until you've finished your reps!*

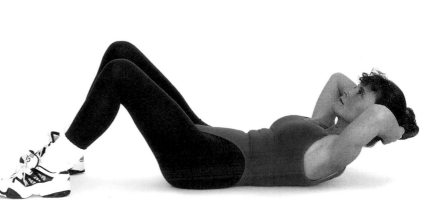

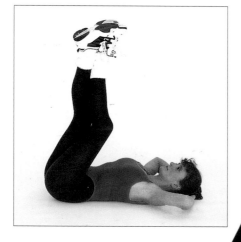

DIAGONAL DOUBLE CURLS

Same start position as previous exercise. Now raise your legs off the floor, keeping knees bent, ankles crossed. Now raise right shoulder off the floor and aim towards your left knee, making two defined movements – lift, one move, across, second move. As you do so, bring legs slightly in to help work the lower abdomen. Return upper body to floor in two moves – *one*, across to centre, *two*, down to floor. Repeat 8 times with right shoulder off floor, eight times with left shoulder.

Hips and Thighs

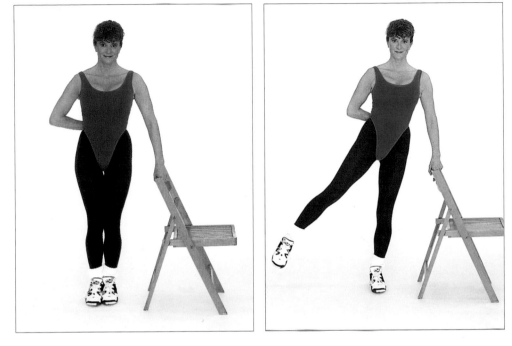

STANDING SIDE LEG RAISES

Stand beside the back of a sturdy dining-type chair, left side on, feet hip-width apart and left hand holding chair back for support. Now, keeping leg straight but knee relaxed, slowly raise right leg out to your right side until you feel the right hip working. Hold for a count of 2, then slowly return to start. Repeat 8 times, then repeat 8 times to other side.

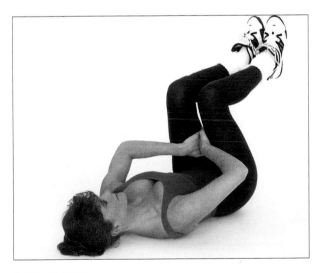

FROG'S-LEG PRESS

Lie on your back with feet together in the air as shown. Place hands on the inner thighs and let knees drop open. Now try to bring knees back together while exerting opposite pressure using palms. Return knees to start. Keep tummy pulled in throughout. Repeat 16 times.

Bottom and Hamstrings

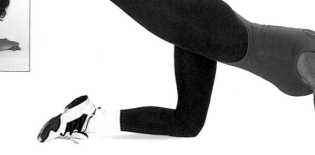

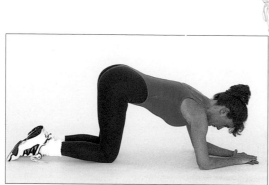

KNEELING LEG RAISES

Kneel on your mat, resting upper body on forearms and keeping tummy pulled in and back strong. Now extend right leg off floor to a lifted straight position as shown, until you feel your right gluteal muscle working, and return to start position. Don't swing the leg, and only lift as high as you need to feel the buttock contract. Repeat 16 times, repeat with left leg.

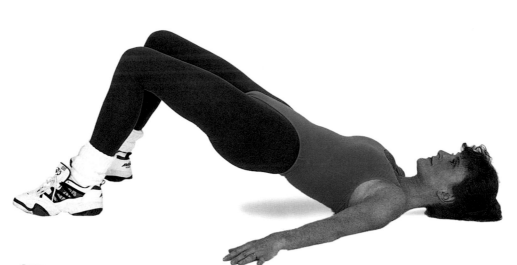

BOTTOM CRUNCHES

Lie on floor with knees slightly bent, arms by your sides and feet flat on floor. Now use your gluteals to raise your pelvis off the floor as far as you can, still keeping your feet flat on the floor. Lower again and repeat 32 times. Concentrate hard on pulling your gluteal muscles in tight to achieve this.

EXERCISE PROFILE

Kay was very uncoordinated in her movements at the start of the programme, and very weak and lacking in confidence in her own ability to improve. She has persisted, however, and towards the end of the ten weeks, her body shape, her fitness level and her muscle tone have improved so much that even we are surprised! 'One of the reasons I gave up smoking was that exercise and cigarettes don't go together. I want healthy lungs now. And I find that regular exercise actually removes the craving for cigarettes, anyway!'

Chest and Upper Arms

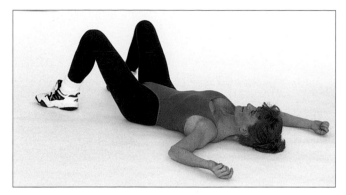

LYING CHEST PRESS

Lie on your back with legs bent, feet flat on floor, tummy tucked in and arms out to either side as shown. Now, with fists closed, bring arms in together until elbows and forearms meet above your chest as shown. Feel your chest and arm muscles working. Lower to start and repeat 16 times. You can use light weights for this exercise in later weeks.

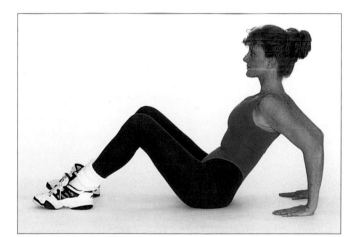

TRICEP DIPS

Sit on the floor with legs bent and arms slightly behind you either side, with fingers pointing forwards, as shown. Now bend elbows and slowly lower upper body towards floor to about 45°. Slowly return to start and repeat the dips 16 times.

Y *ou can lose several years, several pounds and several inches*
   in seconds – just by the way you stand. So here's where we check out
your body alignment – and learn to get it right. Good body alignment – posture – is as important
to the shape and look of your body as is being a reasonable weight or being well toned up.

WORKSHOP 4 # SHAPEWISE 2 – BODY ALIGNMENT

It is a sad fact that nine out of ten women by the time they hit their middle years – and often long before that – have such poor posture that they are adding years to the way they look. Double chins and a protruding stomach are as likely to be caused by pelvic, hip and spine misalignment as by fat. A thick waist isn't just 'middle-aged spread' but a result of years spent sitting incorrectly in office, dining and easy chairs. However, if you re-learn how to sit, stand and walk correctly, with straight shoulders, long neck and pelvis tilted correctly, these problems will be minimized, or even disappear, in time.

Viewed from the side, you can seem to shed pounds just by using your body correctly (see photos opposite). And there are other benefits to 'standing tall', as well. Good posture gives you authority, helps you to look confident, outgoing and in control. People will view you as a more positive person and you will feel so yourself. You will also appear more youthful, as poor posture is associated with old age. Back pain – which plagues most of us at least sometimes – will also be minimized.

Although it is possible to re-align your body in front of a mirror almost instantly, the improvements you make will need re-inforcing by doing some regular body-alignment exercises until that position is completely natural to you. Without this, you may be able to hold the correct position for a minute or two, but your muscles will quickly tire. That is because years of misalignment have caused certain muscles to shorten and tighten, others to lengthen

The Pelvic Tilt

The 'core' of good posture is getting your pelvis into correct alignment, so the first thing to do is practise the 'pelvic tilt' several times a day until it becomes natural to you. Practise by tilting your pelvis first forward (photo 1), then right backwards (photo 3) and finally centre it so that your body is in correct centred alignment (photo 2).

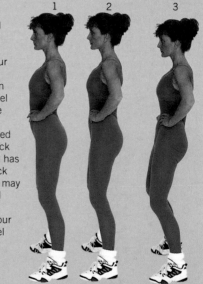

When you are centred correctly, you should have your shoulders relaxed and down, your knees relaxed, your stomach should flatten out and you should feel the base of your spine under your buttocks, which will be contracted slightly. Your lower back will flatten out (Louise has pronounced lower back curve naturally; yours may be flatter). You should also feel your ribcage expand slightly and your chin should be parallel to the floor.

This pelvic position is also the correct one to maintain when you are sitting, walking or lying in bed, and when exercising. Get in the habit of thinking about this correct alignment throughout the day and eventually, with the help of the exercises in this section to back up the new work your muscles are being asked to do, it will become second nature.

and weaken. So you have to exercise to reverse this process and get the muscles back working as they were meant to work.

As an example, if you have rounded shoulders, the muscles of your upper back and backs of shoulders will have lengthened and weakened, while the opposite muscles of your chest and front shoulders will have shortened and tightened. So to correct round shoulders long term you need to strengthen those weak muscles and stretch those short, tight ones. Only when you have done that will the correct posture feel natural to you.

The Total Tone programme in Workshop 3 will go some way towards making these changes but if your posture is really poor you will need extra work. In ten weeks you can achieve a lot, especially if you make a conscious effort all day, every day, to put correct alignment into practice. After all, a few minutes daily exercise won't help much if you spend the remaining 23¾ hours of the day sitting, standing, walking and lying with bad posture. It is these everyday hours that you should use to practise doing everything right.

The exercise suggestions that comprise Workshop 4 are designed to help correct the most usual posture faults that we develop in the middle years (see right). If your figure problems seem to be different from those described here or, indeed, if you want more personal advice on your own body alignment problems, there are several internationally-recognized systems with classes worldwide – check out what you have available in your area. The library, leisure centre or Internet will help you.

● Pilates consists of individually tailored exercise emphasising correct posture and balance (in UK 0171 495 0374).

● The Alexander Technique increases awareness of movement, posture and balance in your daily life (in UK 0171 351 0828).

● Iyengar Yoga teaches total body awareness, breathing and relaxation (in UK 0171 624 3080).

Try The Mirror Test

Photos 1 and 2 show Louise modelling in a classic misaligned pose, typical of a body which has spent years being asked to sit and stand incorrectly and has been under-exercised.
● Habitual slumping over desks and in chairs has weakened and rounded upper back. Head pokes forward.
● Weak stomach muscles and incorrectly aligned pelvis allow stomach to protrude.
● Sway back due to hips incorrectly aligned, tight hip flexors.
● Knees rotated inwards due to weak gluteal (bottom) and outer thigh muscles. Flat feet likely result of this.
● Ribcage slumped, shoulders rounded, resulting in droopy bust-line and shorter, thickened waist.

Photos 3 and 4 show Louise re-aligned correctly, typical of someone aware of the importance of posture and regular exercise to tone, stretch and strengthen muscles. This correct alignment will feel anything but natural to your body if you have had poor posture for years.
● Pelvis tilted correctly (see far left) by contracting gluteals and pulling in tummy immediately gives a slimmer, firmer line to lower body. Abdominal and gluteal exercises needed to maintain this position.
● Knees rotated back out to the correct alignment by tightening gluteals. Foot arches raised. Outer thigh exercises needed to reinforce improvement.
● With a stronger leg and lower body position, back naturally straightens, shoulders relax and come back and down. Back strength exercises (all sections) and chest stretches needed to maintain this posture.
● With shoulders correctly aligned, neck and head sit naturally on spine and waist lengthens.
If you have good posture like that shown above, then you need not do this workshop. If, however, you look more like photos 1 and 2 the exercises that follow, and repeated practising of the pelvic tilt (see left) will improve your posture quickly.

THE BODY ALIGNMENT EXERCISES

Do the exercises as often as you can – you can add them on to your Total Tone programme or fit them in whenever you like – always warm up before exercise and cool down afterwards (if doing alignment exercises separately from the Total Tone, use the Total Tone warm-up and cool-down).

Abdominal strength
Do extra work on the Abdominal Crunches, Diagonal Crunches and Double Crunches that appear on page 40 in the basic Total Tone Exercises, plus the ADD-ONS for Waist and Stomach (see page 44).

Gluteal (buttock) strength.
Do extra work on the Squats, Forward Lunges and Side Leg Raises that appear on pages 38, 39 and 40 in the basic Total Tone Exercises, plus the ADD-ONS for Bottom and Hamstrings (see page 46).

Back strength
Do extra work on the Back Extensions that appear on page 41 in the basic Total Tone Exercises, plus the two exercises pictured here.

Chest stretch
Do extra work on the calf and chest stretch described in the Total Tone Warm-up (page 37), extra work on the cool-down chest stretch in the Total Tone Cool Down (page 42), plus the three stretches described on page 51.

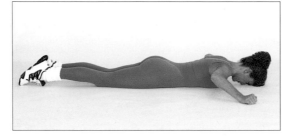

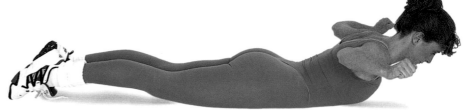

1 LYING EXTENSIONS WITH FLIES
Lie on your stomach with arms out at right angles to the body, knees relaxed. Bring upper body and arms off the floor and, keeping body raised, bring arms out to sides and round to touch bottom. Return to start and repeat 12 times.

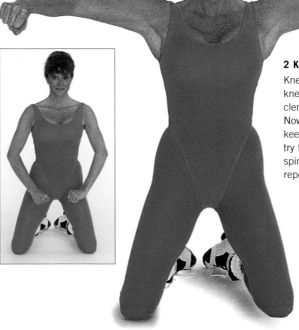

2 KNEELING LATERAL FLIES
Kneel as shown (far left) with knees hip width apart and fists clenched in front of your thighs. Now lift arms up and out to sides, keeping shoulderblades back and try to get them to meet at the spine. Squeeze hard. Relax and repeat 30 times.

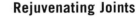

All-day Tips

✔ Think about your body as often as you can. Get into the habit of correcting posture all the time (driving and lying in bed included).

✗ Don't sit with your legs crossed.

✗ Don't stand with weight on one leg.

✗ Don't wear high heels all the time; they encourage poor posture and backache.

✔ Remember that posture faults which have developed over many years will take time to correct – keep going!

✔ Check your office, dining and easy chairs for support. Very many chairs are designed to encourage bad posture. Sit with your lower back supported by the back of the chair – if it is too deep, add firm cushions.

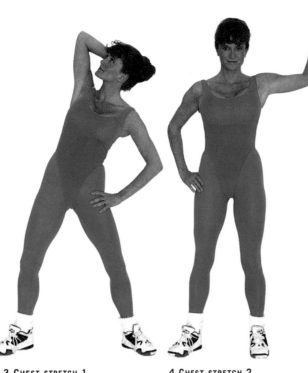

3 CHEST STRETCH 1

Stand as shown, left hand on left thigh, right hand behind head. Bend slightly to the left, keeping back aligned with hips. Feel stretch in right side of chest as you move right elbow back. Hold and then relax. Repeat to other side.

4 CHEST STRETCH 2

Stand left side to wall as shown, forearm and palm touching wall. Feel stretch across chest. Gently move chest forward (moving chest only) and feel stretch increase. Hold then relax. Repeat other side.

Rejuvenating Joints

Several people – even those as young as their mid-forties – have said to me, 'It's too late for me to take up exercise – I feel too stiff and my joints won't take it.' Osteoarthritis (the 'wear and tear' type) can begin at any age, but is more common after the middle years. Most specialists now agree that exercise is beneficial to arthritis sufferers (if it is gentle and done sensibly), and even more important, can help keep arthritis at bay. Stretching exercises help mobility and toning exercises are as important to the arthritis sufferer as they are to anyone else – if not more so! If you have arthritis, your doctor should provide you with suitable exercises and/or refer you to a physiotherapist, and he or she should recommend regular walking (with cushioned shoes and preferably on short grass).
You could show him or her the Total Tone Exercises in this book and see if he thinks they are suitable for you. The stretches that appear in the Total Toning Programme (warm-up and cool-down) are suitable because you take the stretch just as far as you can and no further. But not all 'aches and pains' ARE due to arthritis – they may well be simply the result of inactivity, in which case, check with your doctor that it IS fine to exercise – then begin as soon as possible, taking things at your own pace.
You only have to look at the vast numbers of people of 50, 60, 70-plus at yoga classes, body conditioning classes, aquarobics and so on, to realise that there IS no age at which you have to hang up your trainers and say, 'That's it – I'm too old'. With common sense and motivation, you can improve your body, and help yourself to feel and look better, whatever your age.

5 THE LONG BODY STRETCH

The long body stretch photographed here helps total body posture and is not quite as easy as it looks!
Lie on your back on a mat, arms by sides, legs out straight. Squeeze gluteals, point toes. Elongate waist as far as you can (wriggle your bottom down the floor to achieve this), and raise arms up and over your head until backs of hands are touching the floor (you may not be able to do this, but go as far as you can without arching back). Feel your shoulder and ribcage stretching out, feel your stomach flattening into the floor and breathe deeply and slowly. Hold the stretch for a count of 30, making sure you aren't raising your mid-body section off the floor to try to accommodate the stretch. As you get into the stretch you may find your hand reaching further towards the floor. Come up from the stretch gently by rolling on your side. In time you may want to hold this stretch for 2-3 minutes.

*M*ost of us think that we look after our skin well – but few of us,
despite spending a fortune on face creams and cleansers, actually do.
In this workshop, we sort out the fact from the fiction and get down to the bare
essentials that will really work to make your skin look, and feel, younger.

WORKSHOP 5 BARE ESSENTIALS

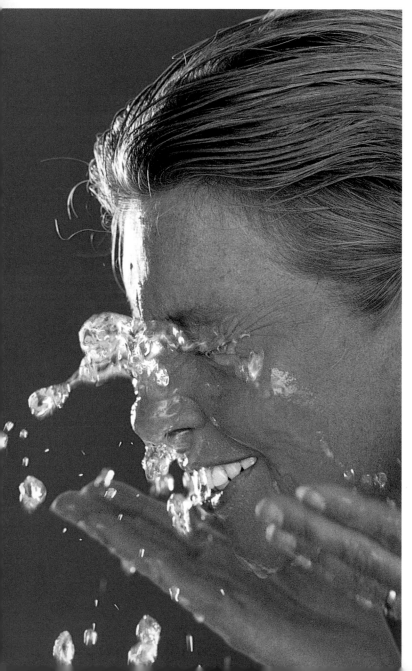

When we think of the ageing face, we usually think first in terms of wrinkles, yet various other factors affect how old your face looks just as much. Bags and sags, coarse skin texture, dull skin tone, dark shadows – all these can age you more than a few 'expression lines' do. True, it is easier to prevent these problems than to cure them but, nevertheless, you shouldn't think that the only way to rejuvenate your face is to fork out for a surgical facelift. Other less drastic strategies can work almost as well as surgery – and sometimes a sight better.

War on wrinkles

Very many factors affect the amount, pattern and depth of wrinkling, and most of these factors are things you can alter. Adopt as many of the following strategies as you can, both for delayed onset of new wrinkles and for diminishing the appearance of the wrinkles you already have.

● Moisturize regularly. Most women over 30 own daytime moisturizer and night cream too – but don't use them properly! To be effective, moisturizers need to be used every morning and night, and with not too mean a hand. If you can't afford to spread plenty of product on your face and neck every single day, then don't buy an expensive cream. I've watched women 'moisturizing' their faces, putting a small dab of cream in the middle of each cheek then trying to make it spread up to the forehead, outsides of eyes, round the chin . . . the very areas that need it most are getting virtually none. So buy a cream with which you can afford to be lavish. (See box 'Which cream for you?', overleaf).

If you buy nothing else, buy a day-time moisturizer that sinks in quickly and can be used as a make-up base, then a more heavy-duty night cream or oil which gets a chance to work while you sleep. A separate eye cream is also a good idea as these are very light to apply and won't have you 'dragging' the delicate skin around your eyes, but this is not essential.

● Water your skin inside and out. Drinking lots of water really does seem to improve the skin's condition, and my own skin benefits very much from a morning spray, before moisturizing, of canned Evian water.

● Relax. A tense face encourages the formation of wrinkles, especially around the outer eyes, bridge of nose and forehead. When people are sleeping peacefully they look much younger – that's because in relaxed sleep all the expression lines are smoothed away. Similarly, if you are happy more than you are miserable or angry, your face will reflect that as you get older. Laughter lines are fine – but frown lines or down lines are not so flattering! If you find it hard to keep your face relaxed, get into the habit of regularly relaxing your jaw and unclenching your teeth, and de-stress the eye area by exerting shiatsu pressure with the middle fingers of each hand just inside each inner eyebrow. Hold the pressure for 20 seconds. Do the same with fingers below outer eye on the edge of the socket bone.

● Give up smoking and avoid smoky atmospheres. There is less oxygen in the bloodstream of smokers and constriction of the capillaries to the skin doesn't allow the full benefit of oxygen and nutrients to the skin.

● Eat a diet high in antioxidants, (such as the diet plans in this book) which 'mop up' the free radicals. The antioxidants are vitamins A, C and E, and the mineral selenium.

● Keep your weight steady and don't get too thin. If your weight constantly yo-yos more than a half stone or so it eventually shows in your skin. Also if you become too thin, your face may lose its natural 'padding' of fat which helps to plump out lines. Lastly, don't lose weight too quickly or, again, wrinkles will be more likely to show.

● Keep the sun off your face. Flying in the face of most expert opinion, I'm a great believer in a little sun being good for the spirit and a great relaxer, and therefore good for the body. I will sit out in the sun in small doses – very well protected by cream – but I NEVER worship the sun with my face. I wear good-quality dark glasses, a hat if necessary, a top factor cream and whatever.

Because the sun will damage the thin layers of skin on your face if you let it, destroying the collagen and elastin fibres of the dermis and encouraging wrinkles, and it will also cause red thread veins. Both UVA and UVB rays are now known to cause premature skin ageing. So treat your face and neck to a twice-weekly tan out of a tube (many brands are now quite brilliant) and keep the sun off your face.

● Check out the weather. 'Weather-beaten' is an expression most of us will recognize and it is very apt. Almost any kind of adverse weather will affect your skin, not just the sun. So protect your skin with moisturizer and make up against the cold and winds. Check out the 'weather' indoors, too – central heating will dry your skin out and cause fine lines. Take an Evian spray to work and spray your face regularly if the atmosphere there is dry, and moisturize, if you can, once during the day.

The best weather for your face? Barely warm – and raining. So walking in the rain is not such a bad thing after all!

Stop the drop

Although we worry so much about wrinkles, in fact I don't believe that they are the main enemy. It is the 'sags and bags' on the face that are so ageing. For instance, eyelids or brows that have dropped, eye bags, and jowly chins or jaw-lines that have lost their definition. The good news is that you can do a great deal to 'stop the drop'.

Here's how:

● Keep a reasonable weight. Avoid 'yo-yo' dieting or losing many stones – the loose skin on your face will be a problem.

● Keep your face well exercised (*see page 55*). People rarely think about the muscles in their faces but, like the body muscles, they need regular toning workouts too.

● Diminish eye bags with a twice-daily eye-pack. Cold used herbal tea bags, slices of cucumber or potato placed on each closed eye for a few minutes will reduce puffiness considerably. You can also buy gels that have a similar effect and which you can leave on under make-up.

Skin condition

Skin texture, tone and condition can all alter as we age. Here are some of the most usual changes that can be expected, with solutions.

Dryness

Dry, flaky, rough patches of skin should improve greatly with your anti-wrinkle routine (see previous pages). If they still persist, try a mild facial scrub, but do make sure it IS very mild – labelled 'for sensitive skin'. Alternatively, 2 to 3 times a week rub a little oatmeal mixed with honey into your face, rinse and moisturize. If your skin isn't at all sensitive, you could also use a mild AHA-containing moisturizer/night cream rather than those suggested left. AHAs exfoliate the top layers of skin, revealing new skin underneath. However, I would never use an AHA cream every day - 3-4 times a week is plenty.

Open pores, blackheads

Far from just a plague of the teen years, open pores can actually get worse around the menopause. Pores need a tricky combination of deep cleansing with fairly gentle treatment. Contrary to what many experts will tell you, skin toning lotions don't close open pores; they simply make the skin feel tauter by their astringent and/or cooling action. If you use a good light cleanser or facial wash, toner isn't really necessary at all, especially if your skin is dry. A spray with Evian, tissued gently off, is all you need to remove any last traces of dirt and leave skin fresh.

Large, blocked pores respond best to three things: exercise, steaming and masks. Your skin is an organ, and needs oxygenating. To oxygenate it properly you need good circulation, which means regular aerobic exercise. By now you should be doing the Stamina programme in Workshop 14, and should see quite immediate improvements in your skin tone. Twice a week, put your cleansed face over a bowl of just-boiled water and keep it there for 2 minutes. Cleanse again and finally put on a refining face mask, just over the open pored areas (see Face Masks, below). Wash off with lukewarm water after 15 minutes and moisturize.

Pallor

As skin gets older it tends to lose pink tones and 'fades'. You can counteract this with enough sleep, a healthy diet containing plenty of vitamins and minerals, and – again - plenty of exercise. Do all you can to improve the circulation to the face, including massage and facial exercises (see right and the self-massage described on page 110). Lastly, stress can cause pallor and dark under-eye circles, so try all the anti-stress treatments described in Workshop 15.

Eyes

I know your eyes aren't skin, but as healthy bright eyes make such a difference to your look - and can take years off you - here are some tips for getting that bright-eyed look. Again, you need enough sleep (but not too much), a diet rich in vitamin C, a life that you enjoy (depression dulls the eyes) and every now and again, before a special occasion, you can use eye drops such as Murine, which clear the eye whites.

Face Masks

Buy or make a face mask to suit your skin. If you have combination skin – say, open pores around the nose or chin, but dry elsewhere, put two different masks on at the same time. *Enriching, moisturizing masks:* mashed avocado, honey and cream; mashed banana mixed with egg yolk; mayonnaise; honey and wheatgerm oil. *Refining masks for oily areas and coarse skin:* egg white and oatmeal; egg white and lemon juice; kaolin, yoghurt and oatmeal.

Almost-free Face-lift

Spend two or three minutes a day exercising the parts of your face
that seem most inclined to drop. Within a few weeks most women notice a real
difference in their appearance as the muscles tone up
and their skin looks tauter.

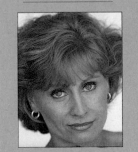
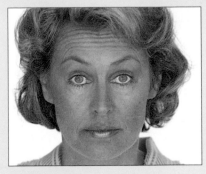

EYEBROW RAISE
Droopy brows make you look tired and sad. Sit with face relaxed, including jaw and teeth, and looking straight ahead. Raise eyebrows up as high as they will go while keeping the rest of your face still. Hold the raise for a count of 5, lower and repeat for 1 minute.

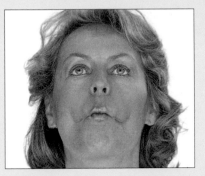

LOWER CHEEK SHAPER
Good if you have little cheek definition. Sit as above, lift chin up and out. Suck your cheeks in as strong as you can for a count of 10. Relax and repeat for 1 minute.

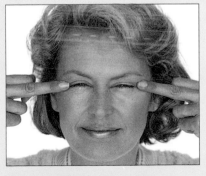

UPPER LID STRENGTHENER
Hooded lids are ageing and 'close up' your eyes. Sit as above. Place middle fingers of both hands on the outer edge of both top lids (feel the bone at the edge of the socket to locate). Keep a medium pressure with the fingers. Now squint lower lids up hard and, as you do so, you'll feel a strong muscle contraction under your fingers. Do this small movement rapidly 10 times, relax, then repeat the 10 pulses plus the relax for 1 minute.

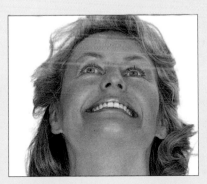

CHIN AND JAW SHAPER
For double chin, jowls, saggy jaw-line. Sit as above. Tilt head back and up slightly. Jut chin out slightly. Open mouth widely by lowering jaw. Now smile as wide as you can and bring back teeth together. Still smiling, lower and raise jaw 10 times slowly. Relax and repeat once more. Feel those muscles working.

Body beautiful

The skin on the rest of your body deserves attention too. Don't forget:

Hands and nails

Use hand cream ALL the time and always wear gloves when you wash dishes or do housework.

Prevent or minimize those brown age spots that sometimes appear on the backs of hands with either a retinol cream or with a hand mask made by mixing lemon juice with avocado. Keep nails smart with a regular manicure – one marvellous benefit of hitting your mid-years is that your nails get stronger and stronger, so make the most of it.

Feet

If you like to go barefoot, make sure your feet are looked after. They respond well to creams, massage and exercise. Hurting feet show on your face, so if you must wear high heels, give your feet plenty of breaks in comfortable footwear.

Lips

Keep well moisturized and protected against the sun with a UVA/B-rich salve or lipstick.

Teeth and gums

Regular visits to the dental hygienist and dentist are a must; as are good food, plenty of vitamin C for healthy gums, scrupulous daily dental hygiene and, if necessary, a whitening tooth-paste for a bright smile.

Body skin

Keep your body skin young by remembering it every now and then! Try the routine here regularly and make sure to use gentle bath oils or creams in the bath or shower.

Relaxing essential oils

Bergamot, chamomile, clary, jasmine, lavender, neroli, sandalwood.

Invigorating essential oils

Basil, cinnamon, lemon, peppermint, pine, rosemary. (Essential oils are available from pharmacies, health food stores and by mail order.)

20-minute Skincare Routine

1 Undress and put on your bath robe. Cleanse face with gentle cleanser to suit skin type, using cotton wool OR use a facial wash.

2 Steam face with head over bowl of just boiled water for 2 minutes.

3 Apply moisturizing, purifying face mask.

4 Bathe (or shower) with a few drops of relaxing (or invigorating, depending upon your needs) essential oil in the bath water. Put used herbal tea bags, or cucumber or potato rings, over your eyes. Relax totally for 10 minutes.

5 Pat body dry with thick warm towels. Apply body lotion all over body while skin is still warm. Take special care of feet, knees, elbows and neck.

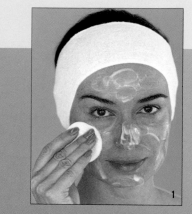

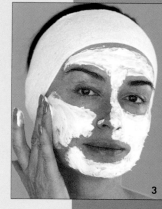

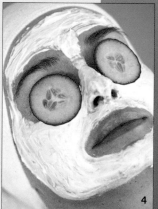

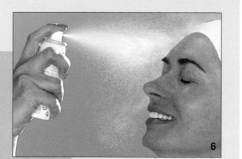

6

6 Remove mask with warm water and spray face with Evian water or splash with mineral water.

7 Apply eye-soothing gel or night eye cream around eyes and on lids (depending on whether you are going out or going to bed).

8 Apply moisturizer if going out, or your favourite night cream/oil to face (I recommend vitamin E oil) if not.

9 Apply hand cream and a nail cream around cuticles

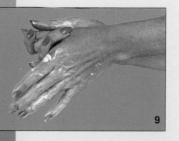

9

5

CELLULITE – WHAT WORKS?

Cellulite is the dimpled fat that appears on many women's lower bodies even if they aren't overweight. It isn't easy to shift but it can be done. Try these strategies and you will see a marked improvement in ten weeks - continue for further improvement.

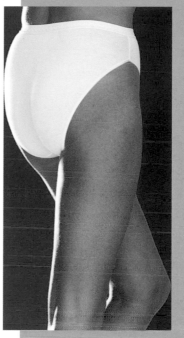

• Take lower-body exercise – the most important single factor in cellulite control. Regular toning, aerobic and stretch work for the legs (such as the routines within your 10-week programme) are essential. The proof? Look at any woman who is at her correct weight and does plenty of lower-body work and you will rarely find cellulite.
• Maintain a correct body weight – yes, it is true that thin women can get cellulite, but if you are overweight with cellulite, the cellulite won't go unless you get down to a reasonable weight.
• Eat healthily – I'm not a believer in the idea that cellulite is caused by toxins trapped in fat cells, but a diet such as the Zest Plan (page 103), rich in antioxidant vitamins and other vitamins and minerals, and with plenty of essential fatty acids, will help your skin maintain optimum condition.
• Massage your cellulite regularly. Many tests have shown that if you massage cellulite using a rough mitt, or similar, and a softening lotion or cream every day for a few weeks, the appearance of the cellulite is improved and diminished. You do have to do it regularly, for several minutes at a time, and you have to do it hard! There are many massage kits available, but you don't need to spend a lot – just buy a loofah mitt and some ordinary body lotion – or dilute a little pure vitamin E oil in some almond oil base and get massaging . . .

*T*he right make-up can take years off you. Conversely, the use of dated techniques, and colours and textures that are wrong for older skin, can put years ON. With the help of top make-up artist Celia Hunter, this workshop shows you how to make the most of YOUR face.

WORKSHOP **6** # MAKE-UP MAGIC

*C*elia says 'As you get older, you need to rethink your look every now and again. So many women stick with the same colours, brands, and types of cosmetics that they have used throughout their adult life. But if you really look at your face, and look at what is now available to buy, you may realize that you are a long way from doing yourself justice with the products you are using and the way you are using them.'

Even with the best skin-care routine possible, as described in Workshop 5, our skin and our colouring do change as we age and the cosmetics that suit a 25-year-old will rarely suit a 45-year-old. Here (right) are the mistakes you may be making:

R e t h i n k i n g   y o u r   l o o k

Too heavy a hand

As our skin shows signs of ageing – uneven patches of colour, thread veins or dark circles, perhaps, as well as fine lines - it is tempting to attempt a cover-up job by piling on ever more thick foundation and powder, or to focus attention on the eyes or lips by increasing the colour and amount of make-up you use there instead.

We've all seen the 'whatever happened to Baby Jane?' syndrome on women of 45-plus, and a pretty sight it isn't. The truth is that a heavy hand when applying make-up isn't flattering at 35, let alone 50 or 60. The general rule is 'less is more', and the older you are, the lighter your hand should be. Particularly – absolutely – do not try to hide wrinkles as if you are Polyfilling cracks in a wall. Luckily, help is at hand for getting maximum disguise of age-related face faults with minimum coverage (see 'Catch Up with Make-up' on page 60).

Making up in poor light

Few women have really decent light in which to make up. And trying to do a good make-up job in the half-light of a gloomy bedroom in mid-winter, for instance, is guaranteed to produce all kinds of mistakes. Daylight will reveal brows badly pencilled-in, blusher applied too heavily, and so on. Don't do it. Invest in a set of stage lights for around your dressing table mirror. In summer, check your make-up by a light window before going out.

Not taking your time

As we get older we need to pay more attention to detail, yet most of us pay less. I reckon it is because we have spent SO many years making our faces up, that we're really a bit bored with the whole thing. AND we think we know that face so well, we can do in 2 minutes what used, in our teens, to take half an hour. And, of course, there is the old guilt thing – there are so many more important things to do than make up, so we rush it. Don't. You need to blend foundation in very well, be scrupulous in dusting off any surplus powder, blend eye-shadow properly, apply thin coats of mascara one after the other; not one thick coat in a glop. You need to pay special attention to applying lip colour.

Think of your face now as a 'new' face, and give it the attention you would give it when making up for the very first time in your teens.

Using wrong colours

Skin changes tone as it ages, and so does hair. In general, we get paler. If we don't change our make-up colours to take account of this change, we'll look harsh and/or drained. For example, I used to wear dark-brown eye-shadow to diminish my slightly protruding eyes and create a socket where none existed. For interest, I tried a similar shade on my eyes the other day - and looked an absolute fright, as if I'd been in the boxing ring and come off worst.

Dark colours are drab on most older faces and black, in particular, is a no-no unless you are very dark-skinned. Throw out your black mascara and black eyeliner; it is honestly no longer what you need.

Vivid colours, too, can be unflattering, hard and draining. You may, for example, be dark-skinned with dark hair and have always enjoyed wearing pillar-box red lipstick and think I am talking nonsense. Well, just try a softer red with a hint of pink or blue or brown in it - I bet you one of them suits you better. Blondes, also, often wear red lipstick, but it's rarely the best option over 40. Ideal colours are neutrals or neutral bases with a colour blended in (often by the manufacturer; you don't need to do this yourself!) in light to mid tones. For more on you and colour, turn to Workshop 9.

Flattering make-up for your face will enhance, not dominate!

Using shimmer and shine

As a general rule, the older you are, the more important it is to avoid shimmer, shine, frost and gloss on your face. Shimmer and frost just draw attention to wrinkles, bags, and crepey skin. The worst mistake of all is frosted eye-shadow on your lids if there is any hint of crepiness in them.

So throw out all such things from your make-up chest and instead go for silky mattes for eyes, lips and face. The new-age cosmetics (see panel 'Catch Up with Make-up', overleaf) can provide exactly the right texture for you, so why not use them?

Old techniques

If you are still drawing in the same old socket lines you did 20 years ago and have never felt able to part with your painted-on eyelashes or your black liner inside your lower lids – you're stuck in a time warp! Use the information in this workshop (and in style magazines, etc.) to update your techniques. You should also avoid: using blusher to try to shape your face; using a foundation several shades darker than your real skin tone to try to look more healthy; using a dark lip-liner and filling in the centre in a pale colour; and other such strange make-up tricks. At 16 you may almost get away with it but – at 45, no.

Not looking at your face as it is now

Because you see your face every day, and because the changes in it happen so gradually, you may not notice them. So you are still using the same tricks you did ages ago; which may well not be the same tricks you need now. So sit in front of a good mirror and make an honest appraisal of what you see. This should take in: shape of face (draw hair back and if you're not sure, draw an outline on the mirror in lipstick around your face); condition and tone of skin (to help you decide on your right foundation and powder); eye type (large, small, deep set, wide apart, etc., etc.); under-eye area (do you have any dark circles, bags, deep wrinkles?) and lips (plump and smooth or thin and wrinkled; balanced top and bottom or unbalanced?), and so on. Write down all your good points and what you consider less good points. With the right make-up you can enhance the good points, which will play down the less good ones. You can also do more to correct those less good points (see the information in the pages that follow in this workshop).

Best of all – take a trip to the cosmetic department store nearest to you, or to a branch of Body Shop, and take as long as you can checking out all the cosmetics on display, trying colours out on yourself and seeing what you like and dislike; what suits and what doesn't. Try out foundations for maximum coverage for minimum depth; try everything you can. It really is the best way to get your own looks up-to-date. Then, take advantage of the free make-over that many cosmetics houses now give. (Body Shop will do a quick or long make-over.) Some are better than others, but you will certainly learn plenty. And if you haven't worn make-up in a while, it's a good way to get your confidence back.

CATCH UP WITH MAKE-UP

In the last few years, the quality of make-up has improved tremendously – colours, textures, cover, durability, ease of application, UV protection – you name it. And the best news is that most of the improvements are of maximum help to older skins. Here are some of the best innovations to allow into your make-up bag:

Light diffusing foundations and powders
'Light diffusion' means that fine lines, skin irregularities and blemishes are much less noticeable. The texture of modern foundations and powders are now also much finer, so you get greater coverage while using less – terrific for older skins. Many foundations now offer UVA and UVB protection and other plusses such as antioxidants.

Concealers A decade or so ago, my concealer was a solid, rock-hard stick that came in two shades, very light or dark, dragged on the skin and was probably even more of an eyesore than whatever it was I was trying to hide - the odd blemish or dark circles under my eyes. Now concealers are great, especially the liquid ones that you apply with your finger or a small applicator.

Corn silk powder If you have coarse skin or an oily T-bar, corn silk powder is wonderful – it is SO fine, it gives great coverage without clogging.

Pick-your-own eye-shadow palettes Various cosmetic houses now supply the empty shadow housing which you fill with two, or sometimes three or more, colours of your choice, thus banishing the need to buy a lot of colours you don't like in a ready-made palette just for the one you do like. Go for two or three shades of the same theme: say, for example, cream, beige and light brown or three shades of grey.

Powder pencils Most older eyebrows get sparser, thinner and the colour fades, and you need to use a colour on them to bring your face back into balance. But again, as you get older, eyebrow pencil can look too harsh and be too obvious. The answer is to use a powder colour on your brows, and you can now buy pencils specifically for the purpose. Otherwise, use a grey or browny matte shadow from your eyeshadow collection.

Eyeliner pens Not for anyone over 35 is the harsh liquid eyeliner that comes with a thickish brush and dries the second you've applied it (too thickly, of course!). If your eyes need a little gentle outlining, buy an eyeliner pen or pencil in a soft brown or grey - some you can blend in before they dry to avoid a hard edge to the line.

Lip pencils With age you tend to get fine lines around your lips, into which lipstick can 'bleed' through the day and which will look, quite frankly, awful. Avoid this by using a lip pencil in a natural shade and filling in (for more on this see the make-overs on our guinea pigs that follow). Body Shop even do a special 'no wander' pencil that avoids lip-bleed altogether.

Lip colourings As someone who hates the 'jammy lip' syndrome, I jump at the new lip colourings which add colour to your face without the jam. I think these suit most older lips very well. A lip pencil will do the same trick if you use it all over rather than just for outline, but may not last as long as a lip colour.

THE 30S

a makeover for Sue

1 Sue's skin didn't need heavy foundation – just a little tinted moisturizer to match her natural skin colour, blended in well with fingers or a damp sponge.
2 A touch of concealer around the eyes and nose hid the few dark shadows that Sue has.
3 Celia applied very fine loose powder with a big brush, all over the foundation, then brushed off any surplus.
4 Eye-shadow was kept simple – a rust-brown Dior powder applied on the lower lid then blended up and out slightly to give the 'hardly there' look.
5 Two thin coats of dark brown mascara finished the eyes.
6 Celia used a touch of pinky-beige blusher on the cheekbones to bring out their natural good shape and to help Sue's eyes to sparkle.
7 To finish, a creamy rose-pink lipstick – no need for lip-liner as Sue has no fine lines around her lips.

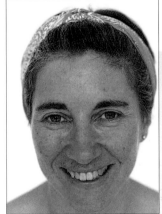

BEFORE:
Sue with no make-up on at all.

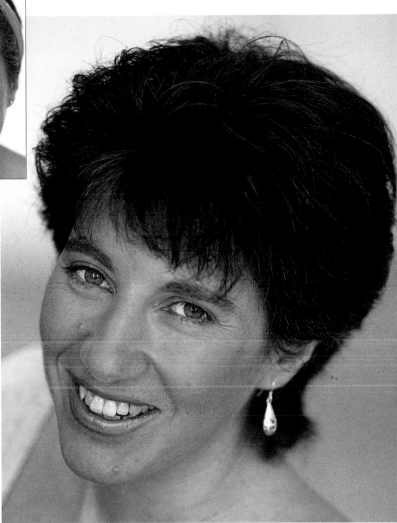

Thirty-nine-year-old Sue normally wears no make-up at all. 'I have never worn it, and don't have any confidence on how to apply it, either.' Celia promised a natural look that Sue could easily copy.

Celia's analysis: 'Sue has a strong, good face with quite high cheek-bones and a nice oval shape. Without make-up, her brows tend to dominate her features and "hide" her very good eyes, which can look greenish, bluish or grey, depending on the light! Her nose is good; maybe slightly long and her mouth is good too, but with a slightly short top lip.

'Sue's skin is neither oily nor dry, and with an even tone and few blemishes. For many women, their 30s can be their skin's best years ever, especially if they suffered from oily skin in the teens and 20s. As long as they moisturize regularly, there may be little sign of wrinkles. Make-up should be slightly more subtle than in the 20s, but skin tone has yet to fade, and so changes can be minimal.'

AFTER
With brows plucked (Celia just thinned them by taking out a few hairs all over) and lips now drawing more attention to her neat, slim jaw-line, Sue's face has really come alive.

Says Celia,
'This is a simple, seven-step make-up that anyone can do in five minutes or so at home.'

Says Sue,
'I feel a completely new person – isn't it amazing what make-up can do?!'

THE 40S

Hilary's new look

BEFORE
Hilary unadorned

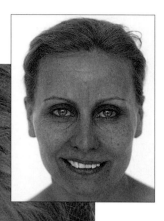

Hilary, 43, has always enjoyed wearing make-up; but now, heading towards her mid-forties, she needs to reconsider her penchant for dark eye-shadows. However, she is sceptical that lighter colours will do anything for her face.

Celia's analysis: 'Hilary has a very good face – quite square but well balanced, with fabulous cheekbones and strong features. Her eyes are lovely – big, blue and expressive, but there's quite a lot of shadowing and darkness around them which we can easily rectify. Her skin and lips can be quite dry without regular deep moisturizing, so I'm going to get as much moisture into her make-up as I can.

'Hilary's skin is typical of her age for someone with fair hair. There are some fine lines around the eyes (which the darker colours are tending to accentuate) and mouth, but no deep wrinkles. She has a few thread veins here and there but not much to worry about. Her skin is sensitive so I'm going to use hypo-allergenic cosmetics and apply them very gently. Be sure to keep your applicators, powder puffs, sponges, etc., washed regularly – make-up, dirt and grease can build up on them which could cause problems.'

AFTER
A glamorous yet soft feel to her make-up has really brought out Hilary's natural beauty.

Says Celia:
'Fair-haired, pale-eyed women – especially over 40 – very rarely look good in dark browns and blacks. As I thought, a lighter touch has enhanced Hilary's looks, rather than detracting from them.'

Says Hilary:
'I'd been using the same make-up colours for years. I'm so glad that Celia has shown me that they were no longer right.'

1 Celia applied hydrating liquid foundation with medium coverage power all over the face, including the eyelids and brow-bone, but using slightly less round the outer eyes and mouth so as to avoid any trace of heaviness there.
2 Concealer was applied to the inner eyes and the under-eye dark circles and on any thread veins all over the face - always use concealer AFTER foundation and before powder.
3 A minimum dusting of ultra-fine loose powder next, just to take any shine off, especially down the nose and on forehead.
4 Celia created a soft eye-liner effect by using a charcoal grey powder eye-shadow, applied along the upper lash line with a small wet brush and blended in to soften.
5 Hilary has a good natural eye socket which Celia enhanced with a soft reddish-brown powder shadow, blended in above and below to soften.
6 Charcoal powder shadow applied lightly under the lower lashes.
7 Celia used brownish-black mascara, with a light hand. 'Avoid lash-building mascaras which can clog; a look you really don't want.'
8 A warm terracotta blusher on the cheekbones lifts Hilary's fair skin and gives her a healthy glow.
9 Lips are outlined with a nearly nude lip pencil from Body Shop and then filled in with a pale clear pink with a hint of peach, then blotted with a tissue to give a more natural finish.

THE 50S

Glamour for Pam

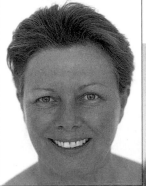

BEFORE:
Pam before her make-up session

As they get older many women try to disguise skin faults and paleness by ladling on more make-up than ever before; which is just what you shouldn't do. Thick foundation clogs wrinkles and makes them seem worse. But you can still look both glamorous and beautiful – as Pam, at 57, shows.

Celia's analysis: 'Pamela has good skin for her age, a little dry with a few broken veins but fine skin quality. By the 50s most women will need to tone their colours down again. Pam's face is a rounded heart shape, and all her features are soft, dainty, delicate. Her current make-up is a bit "stuck in a rut and mumsy" – we need to try more modern colours and products on her to bring her up to date and add a little drama to her softness.

'Around and after menopause, skin texture can change, becoming coarser with open pores, but also with more dry patches. Wrinkles tend to deepen, too. For open pores, I recommend regular use of a face-mask especially for this skin type, but on the open-pored areas only. A mild scrub, like Clinique's for dry skin, is also good. For the dry and/or wrinkled areas, obviously moisturize properly every day and night, and use hydrating cosmetics.

'The best way to make-up wrinkles is to put as little on them as possible – especially laughter lines. So begin blending foundation on to your nose and mid-face area then smooth it to the outer parts of the face so that they receive very little coverage.'

1 Celia used a mid-coverage foundation slightly warmer than Pam's natural skin-tone, applying hardly any to her outer eye area.
2 The foundation was dusted with very fine loose powder and the surplus powder brushed off.
3 Celia applied a medium-brown powder eye-shadow to the socket and corner of Pam's eyes to give her quite heavy lids a lift.
4 A soft coral-pink shadow followed, blended in below the brows and in the centre of lid to give sparkle.
5 A little mid-grey eye-pencil gives definition under the outer edge of the lower lashes.
6 Dark brown mascara, lightly applied to upper and lower lashes, opens up the eyes.
7 Warm pink-toned powder blusher gives a hint of colour to Pam's cheeks.
8 Celia outlined Pam's lips with a lip pencil one shade darker than her natural lip colour, then filled in with a coral cream lipstick and blotted with tissue to finish.

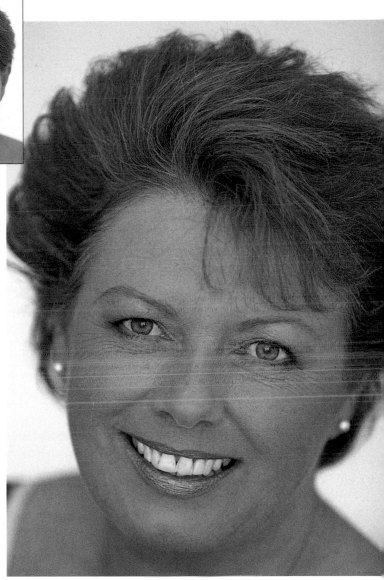

AFTER
Says Celia:
'Well – I have to say, Pam is gorgeous! This shows how small changes can make a big difference.'

Pam's verdict:
'Yes, I do like it. It's more make-up than I'd normally wear, and yet it feels and looks light,'

FACE FURNITURE

Over 40, more women wear glasses (at least some of the time) than don't. Yet we pay little attention to them. The right spectacles should enhance your looks, not send you into a depression every time you put them on.

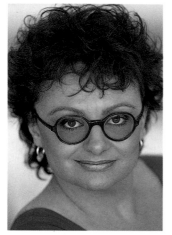

Sal Houston, above, has worn glasses for years and had chosen her heavy and dark-rimmed round specs to go with her dark hair – but they weren't doing her any favours. Says stylist Ceril Campbell, 'Sal doesn't need a disguise, which is what these glasses are. They are hiding her face completely and swamping it, too.' We try some glasses on Sal, below and right, to see what suits her and which are mistakes.

Here's the perfect pair of specs for Sal; they suit her, and her new hairstyle. NOW we can see what you look like, Sally!

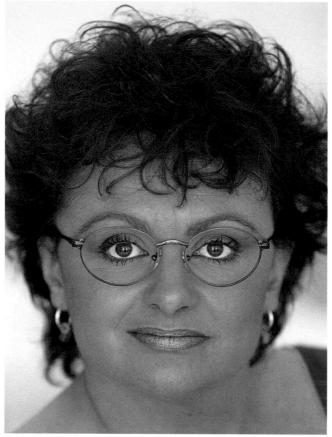

Tips:

- *Buy new frames as often as you can – think of glasses as a fashion accessory (but don't fall for wildly eccentric ones – not everyone may get the joke).*

- *Take into consideration your hairstyle and face shape. Small hair, small face – small glasses! Big hair, big face – big glasses!*

- *Consider your colouring – eyes, skin, hair. Few fair people suit heavy, dark frames.*

- *Don't choose frames in a colour that doesn't suit most of your clothes (unless you're buying several pairs). For example, why buy blue frames if you never wear blue?*

- *Remember your jewellery. If you like to wear silver near your face, don't choose gold frames, and vice-versa.*

- *Try on plenty of frames before deciding – you'll soon realize which frame shapes suit your own face.*

- *Consider contact lenses. Though everyone can look great in the right spectacles, contact lenses – particularly the ones you don't have to remove every night – can be a real confidence boost.*

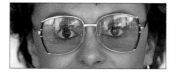

1 These frames are too big and angular for Sal's small face. Her own glasses are a better shape and a rounder frame will soften her squarish jaw-line. Let's try some lighter, oval frames.

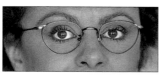

2 These green frames suit Sal well. If you wear glasses all the time, you should consider having more than one pair and changing them to match your outfit or the occasion. If you can't afford to do that, though, best to stick to a neutral colour that suits you well.

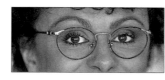

3. These glasses don't suit Sal's face – the tops of the frames should always echo the line of the brow. These are sitting too low.

Quick Tricks for Younger Looks

As the years pass, your face changes. Make-up, as well as all the things you learn in Workshop 5, can help minimize their noticeability.

Heavy jaw: faces tend to 'slip' a bit as the years pass, making the jaw area heavier than it used to be. Minimize this by wearing a strong eye make-up (but not too dark) and blusher to draw attention to the upper part of your face. For evening, you can also shade under the chin and along the jaw line with a powder shader. But do this carefully and don't try it during the daytime.

Small or tired eyes: as we get older, lids tend to sag, causing our eyes to look smaller, and our eyes can get a 'tired' look even when we are not. Help to correct this by choosing a white or cream-coloured soft eye pencil and dot the colour at the inside corner of each eye and blend in well, over foundation and before powdering. Also dot the pencil between upper and lower lashes at the outer corners. If using eyeliner, never take it so that upper and lower lines join at this outer edge – always leave this gap and fill in with the light pencil. Use colours on your lids and use blusher, which always brightens the eyes up.

Thin lips: ageing has the effect of thinning out the lips. If this doesn't suit you, you can make them look larger by taking a lip pencil in a shade barely darker than your own lip colour and outlining the lips just outside (but only just) the natural lip line. Fill in with more lip pencil, then a touch of creamy lipstick. If one lip is thinner than the other, use the same trick but on the thin lip only. You could also use a slightly darker shade on the thicker lip, as dark colours diminish.

Lip bleed: stop lipstick sliding into the fine lines around your mouth by using a lip pencil or a lip tint rather than a creamy or glossy lipstick. If using lipstick, use a long-lasting formula and always blot after applying.

Pale, tired complexion: if exercise, fresh air and sleep don't work, liven up your face with a tiny amount of fake tan and/or a dusting of blusher on the top of the cheeks. Also, choosing eye and lip shades (and clothes) that flatter your colouring will give you a real lift (see 'Colour Confidence' section on page 78).

Tricks not to try . . .

some things it is best to leave rather than try to conceal or correct:

Celia says, 'Even for the camera, I never use shaders to try to correct face shapes. It is so easy for everyone else to see what you've been trying to do that it draws more attention to the "problem". Unless you are a professional, it is very hard to achieve a natural result. That's why I won't do it on my makeovers – I don't like to do anything that a woman can't copy at home.'

The best solution to problems such as saggy eyelids, eye bags, nose-to-mouth lines and poor chin definition is facial exercises (see page 55). Done daily they do bring results.

TOP TEN WAYS TO TAKE YEARS OFF YOUR FACE INSTANTLY

❶ Use blusher.

❷ Get enough sleep and exercise.

❸ Pluck and colour your eyebrows.

❹ Wear a pair of flattering earrings.

❺ Wear less foundation and powder.

❻ Pick a flattering hairstyle (see Workshop 7).

❼ Put a couple of drops of Murine or similar in your eyes.

❽ Wear make-up colours that suit your skin, hair and eye colouring (see Workshop 9).

❾ Make sure your glasses are up-to-date.

❿ Smile.

*I*n this workshop, I've enlisted the help of leading hairdresser Paul Edmonds. Paul, who cut and styled all our models' hair and provided much of the advice that appears in this workshop, appears regularly on TV style shows; he styles for movies and counts top models, actors and TV personalities among his many famous clients. He also has his own range of aromatherapy hair products. For all this, Paul has the most common-sensical approach I have found in any hairdresser – he has a perfect instinct for understanding what style will suit a woman and her hair type, and also recognizes that most of us can't afford the time or money to spend hours on our hair. So read on with confidence, and get the inspiration you need . . .

WORKSHOP **7** # HAIR-FLAIR 1 – SUPERSTYLES

Four Top Hair Swaps to Take Off Years

Whether you want you hair long, medium or short, straight or curly, there's a right and a wrong way to do it! In our 'befores' and 'afters' sometimes the difference is only very small – but the result is wonderful.

GOOD-BYE TO CURTAINS!

Kay is 48 but still wants to wear her hair long. No problem. Says Paul, 'You can wear your hair long at almost any age, as long as it is in good condition and well styled. But you have to be careful – avoid the "curtain effect" of straight sides (see below left) which drags the face down, and long hair will often create a "flat-top" effect because of the sheer weight of it – there is no lift at the roots.'

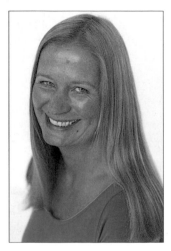

SWAP: Paul has taken a few inches off Kay's hair and graduated the sides. Before drying, he applied Phytovolume for fine, limp hair and then Kay bent forward so that he could blow-dry to give the hair lift. 'Kay is narrow at the temple, with a wide jaw, so we need to finish the style by lifting the hair at the temple and slightly turning the graduated end in to the face.'
The result – a stunning transformation which Kay loves and will have no problem re-creating at home. All she needs is a trim every eight weeks.

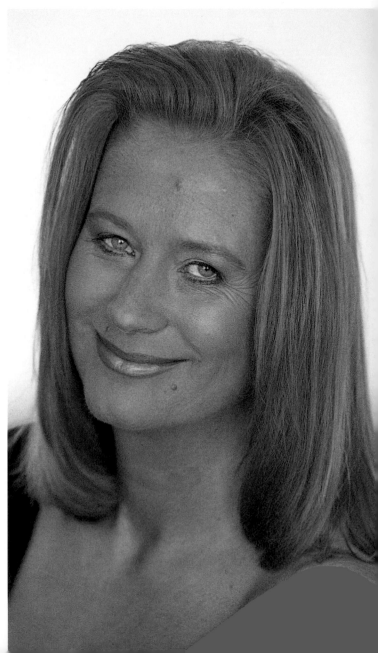

TAKING IT UP

Swap your look in a minute! For a truly instant facelift, pile long hair on top of your head. Angela, 40, has a very thick head of hair that she wants to leave long. Again, however, the 'curtain effect' and hard forehead line are accentuating her oblong face and doing her no favours. When you think of youthful flattering hair, think of 'height and light'.

SWAP: Paul trimmed, conditioned and coloured Angela's hair (see page 72) but agreed that she would look terrific with it piled high. The quickest and easiest way to put hair up is to lean forward, brush all the hair forward, grab it on the crown and put it through a scrunchie. Leave the ends loose or twist them around and secure with pins. Pull some strands of hair out around your hairline to soften the effect and you have a look that you can wear anywhere.

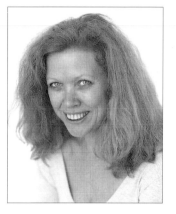

LENGTH WITH LIFT

A medium-to-long layered look is good for most faces and a good halfway house between long hair like Kay's and short. But most women tend to wear this style too heavy – again, producing a 'flat top' effect and bushy sides that don't flatter. Linda, 47, has a very attractive face but her nice eyes and bone structure are being diminished by too much floppy hair. 'I tend to use heated rollers every day otherwise it looks a mess,' she says. And says Paul, 'The top doesn't gel with the bottom; it's a bit too long at the sides for Linda's face, and it's too curly and slightly old-fashioned – heated rollers tend to give this effect unless you are very careful.'

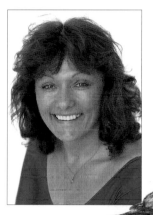

SWAP: Paul has taken the weight off the sides and cut into the top and fringe more to give a more flattering, lighter look to Linda's hair. From the back, however, the length looks exactly the same as it did before. Paul has blow-dried using a round brush to create a soft, wispy, feathered look and Linda is going to try this at home now and banish those heated rollers.

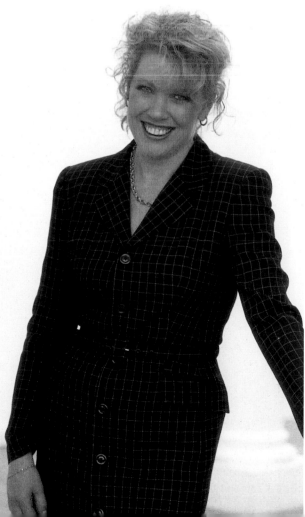

GOING FOR THE CHOP

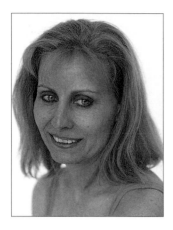

Hilary, 43, has very nice fair hair which she's been wearing in a shoulder-length bob for years. Paul says, 'This style is rather limp and heavy, and manages to make Hilary's lovely face rather un-noticeable. We want a strong style that will complement her strong features. We need to focus the impact on her eyes and cheekbones.

'Yes, it's a brave woman who will go for a short style after years of having it long or mid length - but I'm going to leave plenty of length through Hilary's hair on top so that it won't be that much of a shock! She has very full, naturally curly hair which will hold a style very well if I shorten the length round the sides and blend it in to the longer hair on top.'

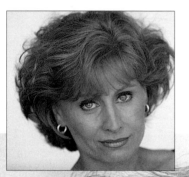

SWAP Hilary's new style works perfectly – and it looks just as good from the side as it does from the front. The side-swept, feathered fringe softens the whole look.

THE INSTANT-FACELIFT HAIR CODE

● Don't keep too much weight below jaw level.

● Think 'light and height' – go for feathered layers and more hair on top of the head than below it.

● Avoid 'curtains'.

● Avoid flatness on the crown – think 'body'.

● Don't scrape hair back severely off the face – keep it quite soft.

● A light and layered fringe almost always looks better than a blunt, heavy one.

● Think 'uplift' – hair brushed upwards (like Pamela's, over-leaf) is always more flattering than hair going downwards.

● Lighten the colour around the face (*see Workshop 8*).

New Looks for Old

– a potpourri of ideas to help you make the most of your hair

Things to be wary of . . .

• Perms: 'Grannie bubbles' are unflattering and a real age giveaway. If you really do need a perm to give body to fine, thin hair, make sure it is a soft one and that the hairdresser avoids the 'bubble' effect at all cost. Pamela's hair had been frequently permed after being cut quite short and this meant that at the crown you could easily see her scalp where the hair fell away into sections. We persuaded her to grow it out (see overleaf) and then, with Paul's clever cutting and straight styling, it looked much more up-to-date.

• The 'set' look. Don't let any hairdresser set your hairstyle into a rock-hard helmet. Up-to-date hair needs to have movement.

• The same style if you've had it more than five years. Paul says, 'People like to stay within their own comfort zone, and this often means sticking with the same old style. Often, just a very slight change in the way it is cut and/or styled can update your hair. Time-warp hair is very ageing. Women tend to keep up with hair trends in their teens and 20s, then at 30-plus, stick with the same old thing. If your style can be dated by other people - then so can you!'
'Also, your style may no longer suit you. Take a good long look at your face and ask yourself if you couldn't do better. Few people suit just one style throughout their lives.'

• Keeping hair long at all costs. Long hair can suit older women, but it needs to be very well looked after, and be thick and glossy and sleek. Long scruffy, 'student' hair on a woman of 40 or 50 will have people sniggering, not admiring.

Choosing a new style

1 Use Paul's guidelines on the previous three pages.

2 Look at hair magazines and cut out styles you like.

3 Look at other women's hair and if you see someone with a style you love, ask her where she got it cut and the name of the stylist. Go there.

4 Talk with the hairdresser; tell him or her what look you'd like and show photos if you can. Be prepared for the hairdresser to adapt this look, or perhaps even tell you it won't suit your hair type. For example, Kay's hair (page 66) would never cut and style like Hilary's hair; it is far too fine and floppy.

5 Remember you've got to style your hair at home, so don't go for anything you will find difficult to look after.

6 Discuss your face shape with your hairdresser and try to choose a style that will suit it. If your face is long and thin, go for a short style with width at the sides, for example. A round face (see Pamela's 'after' photo overleaf) looks best with short hair given body on top. A square or oblong face needs softening with hair wisps around the face and curved (perhaps flicked up) lines, softly layered - even an inch or two of layering cut into the bottom may be enough

7 Your head shape is also important – a style with body can disguise a flat head, for example. Wash your hair and use two mirrors to view your head from all angles.

For information on colouring and conditioning products, see next Workshop.

GET UP-TO-DATE WITH STYLING AIDS

If you've bought nothing but shampoo and conditioner for years you'll be amazed at the quantity of styling product and tools on the market now. Not all live up to their promises, but many are very valuable additions to your dressing table.

Almost any style your hairdresser gives you will be easy to copy at home using the right items. When having your hair cut and styled, make sure to keep asking questions about the right products for you – do you need mousse, gel, anti-frizz spray, serum, volumizing cream, or what?

Will you be able to style just with a normal drier and brush, or not? What type of brush is best for your hair? Round ones produce easy lift and wave; brushes with plenty of space between the 'bristles' are best for thick, long hair. You may need tongs, or a drying styler with its own brush attachment, leaving one hand free to help the style along. You may need a diffuser.

A good hairdresser won't try to persuade you to buy lots of products you don't need, but as hair gets older it often needs some help in order to hold a style.

So you've got the style right – but what kind of condition is your hair in? And could it do with a colour change or enhancement? If you're going grey, what is the best course of action? In this workshop, with the help of Paul and his colourist Tracey, we find the answers.

8 HAIR-FLAIR 2
COLOUR AND CONDITION

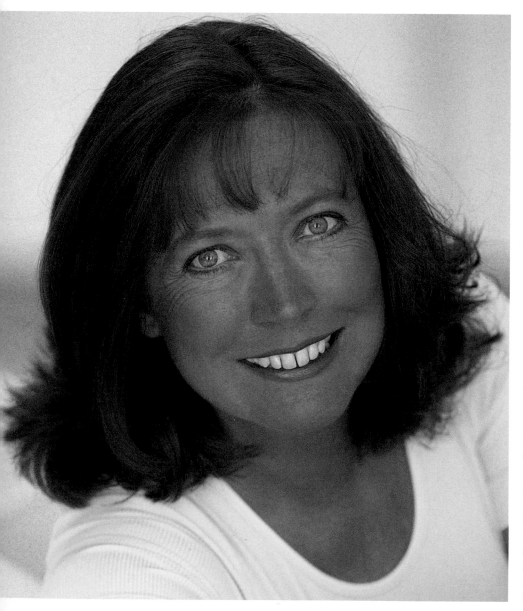

Natural colour that's faded:

Don't feel somehow that you are 'selling out' if you do decide to get your hair coloured after years of leaving it natural. It's really no more of a 'cheat' than wearing make-up or having your teeth fixed! After years basking in being fortunate enough to have a thick head of natural chestnut hair, I took the plunge for the first time recently when I realized I was no longer chestnut but more of a nondescript brown. It took me two seconds to get over the shock and now I'm really pleased.

Also don't worry that your hair may turn a nasty shade of bright orange, or something. Go to a reputable colourist – again, personal recommendation is the best idea. If anything is slightly wrong, it can easily be corrected. If you opt for a semi-permanent colour at first, as opposed to a permanent, this will wash out after about ten washes anyway.

Most women whose hair colour has naturally faded will want to return to their original colour. If you were very dark-haired, you could take this opportunity to choose a slightly lighter shade. Very dark hair can often be 'too much' as you get older – your skin colour changes, your make-up should be softer, and so should your hair.

TIME FOR A COLOUR CHANGE?

Your hair and your looks may benefit from a change of colour if you fit into any of the following categories:

- Natural colour that's faded.

- You've been colouring your hair for ages but wonder if the old colour now suits you.

- Dull hair or a general feeling that you need 'brightening up'.

- Various degrees of grey.

You've been colouring your hair for ages:

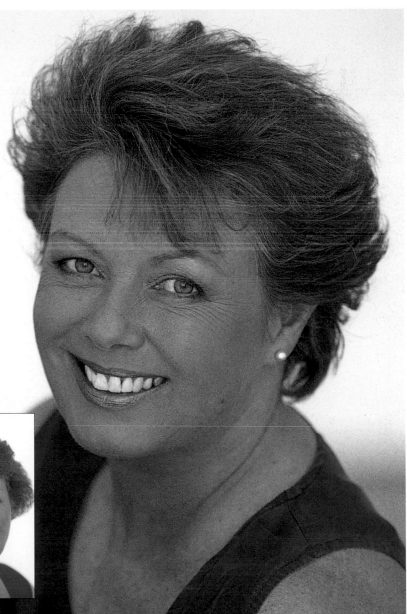

As with hair style, a good hair colour as you get older is one that has the effect of 'lightening" your face. Looks that aren't always ideal, then, are a too-solid, too dark or too harsh colour. What suited you five years ago may not suit you now.

Pamela had been having a straight golden blonde permanent colour on her hair for years, which looked quite solid and lacked light. 'My natural colour was mousy, but I expect I am quite grey now; not that I'd know as I haven't seen my real hair colour in ages!' she said. Paul and Tracey explained that a much more flattering effect would be achieved by using three different colours all through her hair in complementing shades. Pam was dubious – 'I don't want to end up like a tabby cat!' she said.

Little over an hour later, she was delight-ed. Tracey had used rich gold, light gold and a dark gold applied in thick bands of colour. The finished effect is very natural and quite stunning.

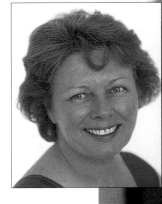

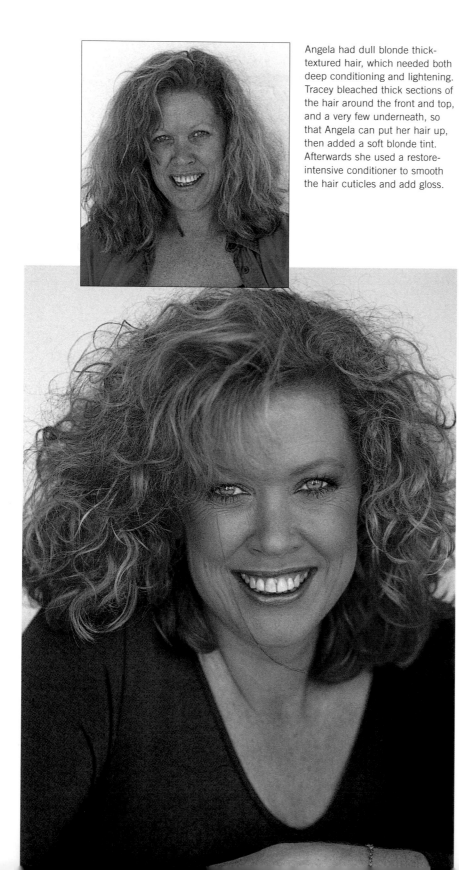

Angela had dull blonde thick-textured hair, which needed both deep conditioning and lightening. Tracey bleached thick sections of the hair around the front and top, and a very few underneath, so that Angela can put her hair up, then added a soft blonde tint. Afterwards she used a restore-intensive conditioner to smooth the hair cuticles and add gloss.

D u l l   h a i r   o r   a   g e n e r a l   f e e l i n g   t h a t   y o u   n e e d   ' b r i g h t e n i n g   u p ' :

Dull hair can be partly rectified by proper conditioning (see page 75) but it can also be changed with colour. The tips we gave for faded hair will apply to you but you can also consider adding just a hint of colour with vegetable dyes, which wash out in a few washes – or, indeed, the shampoo-in temporary colorants which you can buy in the high street and do yourself. These will add shine and a hint of colour which washed out in 2-3 shampoos (unless you use them every shampoo, in which case the colour tends to build up).

You should also consider low-lights – adding deep colours in streaks, highlights, which Tracey did for Angela, or 'tips', which she did for Sal. Highlights added to dark blonde to mid-brown or mousy hair can be very effective, producing that 'light and airy' look that takes off years.

Sal's hair carried a permanent reddish-brown tint which was looking lifeless. Tracey decided to liven up the hair around the face by tipping. She bleached just the tips of the hair and then added an auburn vegetable dye over the whole of the hair, including over the bleached tips – the result is a glossier redder colour on most of the hair, but it is paler at the ends.

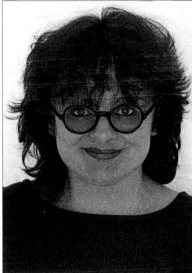

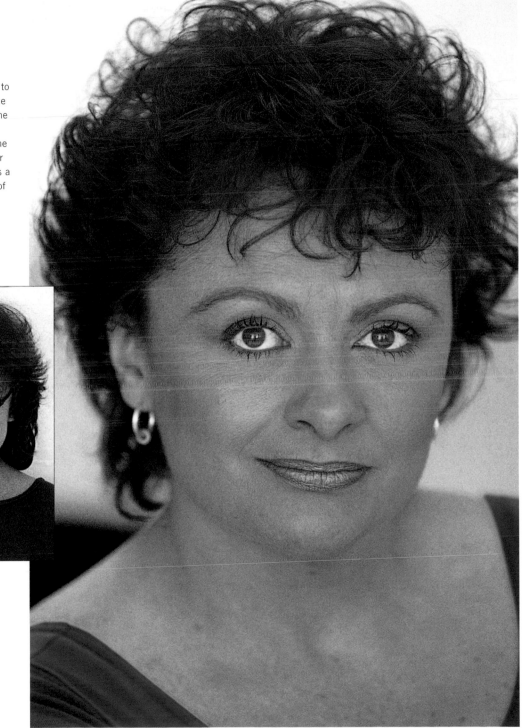

Various Degrees of Grey

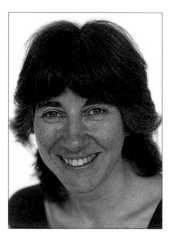

Some women suit grey hair and if you are one of those, it is fine to leave it – particularly if you take care to keep it in tip-top condition because, as Paul points out, grey hair is often dull and without shine.

'Grey hair isn't actually grey at all,' says Paul. 'It is white - but because it is mixed with the darker hair that still contains pigment, it looks grey. One reason grey hair can look all right is because as we get older and our skin colour becomes paler, the lighter, grey colour suits our skin tones better.

'However, I'd say that 80 per cent of the time, it is best to colour it. But I would very rarely do a solid colour on its own -

I'd add colour and then highlights afterwards, which can be very subtle. If someone has gone grey, I would also use a light-to-warm colour – not a dark one.'

Most women who notice their first grey hairs in their 30s or 40s, appearing in their otherwise nicely coloured hair, tend to leave it alone, or cover it with a semi-permanent to match their own colour. But, the more grey that appears, the less successful this will be.

Sue (left) is 39 and had quite a lot of grey hair at the sides but virtually none on top or at the back. Even after cutting, her 'side panels' of grey were still apparent and she wanted rid of them - but didn't want a permanent colour all over her nearly-black hair. The answer was simple – Tracey just used a permanent colour, in dark brown, on those side panels and left the rest well alone – apart from a reddish wash-out vegetable dye to add gloss to Sue's quite dull hair. Sue was extremely pleased with the result.

If you have a lot of grey hair and want a change but nothing too drastic, choose a pale colour or, preferably, two or three colours mixed as Tracey did for Pamela (see page 71).

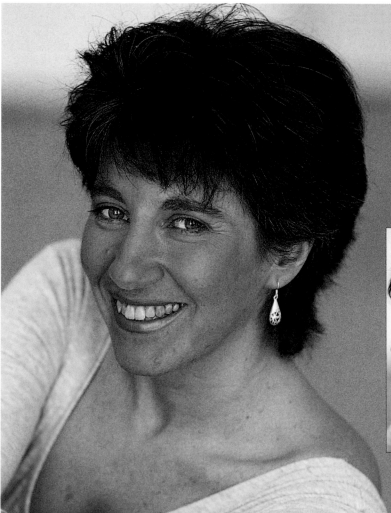

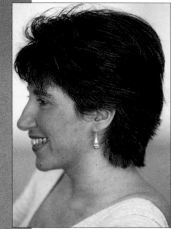

CONDITION UPDATE

**Whatever your age and the current state of your hair, it shouldn't be difficult to get it in good condition
and keep it that way. Here are the solutions to the most frequently asked hair condition questions.**

Q My hair is oily at the scalp and dry at the ends. Is there a conditioner to deal with both problems at once?

A There are some that claim to condition only where it is needed, but in my experience the best solution is to simply condition the ends of the hair and leave the roots alone. Also, get trimmed regularly to chop off those dry ends.

Q Is there such a thing as product build-up on hair and what should I do about it?

A If you use a lot of leave-in conditioners, mousses, etc., obviously there will be build-up on the hair. When you wash your hair, they will be removed. Some shampoos claim specifically to remove 'build-up', but any shampoo should do the trick.

Q Can your hair get used to certain shampoos, conditioners, etc., so that they work less well after a time?

A Some experts say 'yes', others say 'no'. The sensible solution is simply if your usual products are working well, then continue with them. But if your hair is being difficult, dry, over-oily, frizzy, or whatever, for no reason you can work out, having read all of this page, then by all means try something new (trial-size first). Hair does change and you can't expect to go on using the same old products forever with the same results.

Q Can my diet affect my hair condition?

A Yes – a healthy diet like the Zest Plan (page 103) will give hair its best chance of being healthy too. You need enough protein, vitamins, minerals and essential fatty acids in your diet. Many women report better hair condition when they have been taking evening primrose or starflower oil for a while. Poor diet can lead to dull, dry, brittle hair.

Q Can heat affect hair condition?

A Yes - electrical hair tools if used too often and at too high a heat, too close to the hair, will dry it out and cause split ends. The answer is to use them with caution. Keep the hairdryer at least 8 inches away from your hair and use blow-dry lotion or leave-in conditioner. Use heated rollers sparingly and buy some of the new ones that have a low heat setting.

Q My hair's been in bad condition since I began regular swimming. What can I do?

A Chlorine will strip moisture from your hair, as will the sea, bleach, and even the sun. You can buy pre-swim conditioner which you apply to your hair thickly and it forms a barrier while you swim (I agree that swimming caps are not the most elegant or comfortable of things). In fact, any thick cream conditioner will do this job, though if you're in the water long enough, eventually it will wear off. After swimming, rinse and wash hair straight away and use an intensive conditioner. You can buy brands specially to counteract the effect of chlorine – Ultraswim is one. A weekly deep conditioning treatment (wrap your hair in a hot towel to help it work) is also a good idea.

Q Any solution for frizzy hair that I want to look sleek?

A After shampooing, condition it thoroughly then rinse and use an anti-frizz styling lotion such as Phytologie Hair Straightening Balm or Frizz-Ease while blow-drying with a heated styling brush on LOW, using your free hand to keep smoothing the hair down as you dry. Also try hair serum – a little of this non-greasy lotion goes a long way.

Q My hair has become more coarse over the last year or two. I am 48. Why is this?

A Hair does tend to become more coarse in some women. Others find it thins and becomes finer. Hormonal changes around the menopause are the most likely answer. For coarse hair the only thing you can practically do is make sure to keep it very well conditioned to keep it supple and give it shine. Fine, thinning, limp or floppy hair will benefit from correct cutting (short hair generally looks best), and the use of volumizers or mousse when styling.

Q Which is the best moisturizer for dry hair?

A Almost impossible to answer. But certainly, you don't have to spend a fortune. Like face creams, it is more important to use a conditioner regularly, use enough to cover all your hair (unless you're not conditioning the roots) and follow the instructions. Conditioner also works better in a warm atmosphere. It's a case of trying trial-size or sachet conditioners until you find one that really suits your hair. Or, if your hair condition is brilliant after you've been to the hairdresser, you could purchase the products they used, which are usually available to buy. Another idea is to make your own conditioner – egg yolk, mayonnaise or even neat warmed olive or walnut oil will work (but be careful to rinse it off well). For oily, limp hair, beer works well.

C eril Campbell is one of the UK's top style counsellors. She makes over presenters for the BBC, has her own style slot on Sky TV and has helped countless TV viewers and magazine readers to find their own best looks. Ceril had great fun persuading our 10-week participants to rethink their clothes for Workshops 9 and 10. The results speak for themselves …

WORKSHOP **9** # STYLE ASSESSMENT 1
FINDING YOUR OWN STYLE

What you wear has an enormous bearing upon how you feel, how young you appear, and upon how others think of you. Yet almost all of us – at least some of the time – don't get our clothes right.

Here are some of the reasons that are most often quoted: 'I've no time to shop for clothes', 'I can't afford expensive clothes, or lots of them', 'It doesn't really matter what I wear anymore', and 'I'm hopeless at choosing clothes for myself; I've got a wardrobe full of mistakes so I'd rather wear what I feel comfortable with', 'I'm not sure of the right "look" now I'm middle-aged; fashion is for the young'.

In truth, you CAN get away with a lot at 25 that you can't at 50, but that is no reason to just give up and decide to live (and maybe die) in leggings and baggy jumpers, or per-haps to get into the frumpy grannie look once past 40.

This workshop is all about finding your own style. Using our 10-week participants as models, we help you to choose the right colour for you, the right look for particular occasions, discuss how much notice you should take of the current fashions, and show how to update your wardrobe without spending a fortune.

Finding your new look

If you've lost some weight, toned yourself up, treated yourself to a new hair-do – don't spoil everything by carrying on in the same mumsy skirts and tops; or tatty jeans and sweatshirts. Now is the time to treat yourself to some new clothes. But first, before you rush out to start buying, you need to consider some factors. They will help to prevent you from the buying disasters you've undoubtedly had in the past!

Says Ceril, 'The first thing to consider is what you actually WANT from your clothes. For all of us the first priority is to fit our clothes to our lifestyle. As an extreme example, I've known women blow a hard-earned £500 on a high-fashion ball-gown they will wear only once, and then feel guilty about buying decent casual clothes that they could wear every weekend.'

So, RULE ONE – think hard before buying any item. Will you get value out of it? Does it fit in with the way you *really* live?

'Next,' says Ceril, 'Consider what you look good in. The pages that follow give you advice on choosing the right colours, styles and materials for you, and Workshop 10 shows how to dress to flatter your body. So make sure anything you buy fits these simple criteria.'

'Then you need to ask yourself, "Is it easy to wear?", because anything you don't feel comfortable in is unlikely to be worn often – so move around in the garment, watch yourself sit in it, walk in it. Is it a good fit? Raise your arms over your head in it.'

'If you feel it "wears easy" then you'll enjoy wearing it.'

'It will also help if what you choose will team with other things in your existing wardrobe (unless you really are starting from scratch, in which case you still need to buy things that can be mixed and matched). Often really nice garments remain unworn simply because they don't fit in well with what you already have, and that includes accessories. If choosing a colour that's a new one for you, bear this in mind.'

If you follow all these criteria you are unlikely to need to worry too much about whether an outfit is the right one for your age. But just in case you're still not sure, on pages 81 and 82 we consider if there is such a thing as an unsuitable look for an age, and we debate just how much of a slave to the current fashion trends you should be.

Creating the right image for yourself is as much about thought, balance and confidence as it is about money and time.

Colour Confidence

Find your season and seasonal colours, and see over for how to use this information

SUMMER

Summer skin has pinky blue undertones. Usually fair and pale with hair ranging from very blonde to ash or brown, with auburn tones or grey. Eyes are soft greyish or pale.

Summer colours – all pastel pinks and blue pinks, raspberry, blue reds, burgundy, maroon, light lemon-yellow, plum, lavender, mauve, soft white, rose-beige, light-to-medium blue-greys, roe-brown, greyed navy, clear or grey-toned blue, aqua, bluey-greens.
NO orange, gold, black.

WINTER

Winter skin also has pinky blue undertones. Most winters are dark-haired and have greyish-beige or sallow complexions. Winter eyes have more contrast between the white and irises than summer eyes.

Winter colours – mostly clear bright colours, light and dark-blue-toned pinks, clear and bright reds, blue-toned reds, clear yellows, royal purple, icy violet, white, taupe, grey, black, navy, bright blue and ice-blue, bright turquoise, clear bright greens.
NO orange, gold.

SPRING

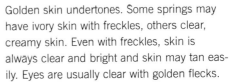

Golden skin undertones. Some springs may have ivory skin with freckles, others clear, creamy skin. Even with freckles, skin is always clear and bright and skin may tan easily. Eyes are usually clear with golden flecks.

Spring colours – light oranges, apricot, peach, salmon, all corals, light rust, peachy pinks, clear and orangey reds, clear gold, golden-yellow, violet, ivory, creamy beige, camel, light warm grey, golden-brown, tan, light clear navy, most clear blues, turquoise and aqua, clear pastel to bright-yellow greens.
NO black, burgundy.

AUTUMN

Golden skin undertones, with red or auburn hair, with freckled, fair, ruddy or dark golden skin. Autumns with pale eyes will look better in the muted autumn colours.

Autumn colours – all oranges, deep peach, salmon, rust, terracotta, orangey and dark reds, gold, yellowy gold, creamy gold, goldy beige, camel, all browns, blue, turquoise, greens.
NO pink, burgundy, purple, grey, black.

COLOUR CONFIDENCE

– or life beyond black leggings...

So you're in a clothes rut. Because it's easy, you always opt for black (or another dark neutral colour) and, because it's easy, you opt for leggings and a top. With the help of participants Angela, Sal, Hilary and Linda, we look at some more flattering alternatives.

When you put on an outfit in a colour that suits you, a wonderful thing happens – you look better. . . you look younger. . . you even look healthier. . . your skin-tone comes alive. . . and your eyes sparkle. When you put a colour near your face that DOESN'T suit you, the reverse happens. So – what suits YOU?

You reckon black suits you – after all, it's slimming, isn't it? And it always has suited you, hasn't it? Well, sadly, black is one of the few colours that suits VERY few older women indeed. Yes, you may look slim and smart in it – but over 40 it will rarely be doing you any other favours. And there are more flattering colours for you that will also make you look slim and smart.

To find your own best colours, try the 'season' test. Ceril explains, 'Although it isn't an exact science, most of us can be categorized into one of the four "seasons", depending upon the colour and tone of our hair, eyes, and skin (see previous page). See if you can work out which season you are. Find a selection of materials in the colours that fit into the category you think you may be and hold them up to your face. If the colours bring your face alive, then you are that season. Most people can wear colours from other seasons and some may look all right. Indeed some people are a mix of more than one season, but this system is a good starting point. Within your colour season, you will find some colours that you prefer to others, and preference is, of course, important. You can wear colours outside your season (even black!) if you wear them with one of your own colours near your face.'

Pale turquoisey blue is one of Sal's really good colours – her face sparkles and her eyes really stand out.

Sal, a winter, has always worn virtually nothing but black. She will look her best in clear bright and icy colours, although she *can* wear black as she has dark eyes and hair.

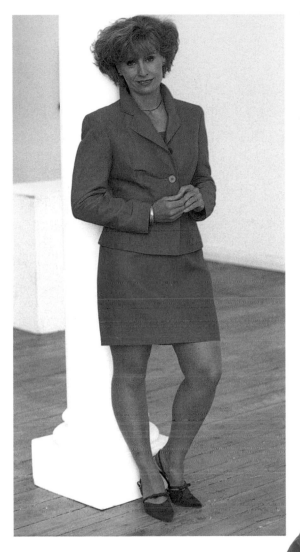

Hilary is a 'spring', but tends to live in drab browns and rarely wears bright colours. The moment we put this coral suit on her she looked fantastic and her personality began to bubble, too. This is one of spring's best colours.

Angela is a spring, and like Sal, loves wearing black. Well, she still can wear black, but if she teams black trousers with an ivory top, like this jacket, she looks 100 per cent better. Ivory or cream are better than white on a spring.

CASUAL CHIC

Over the last ten years, leggings have changed from being the streetwise uniform of teenagers to the definitely unchic uniform of sloppy middle-aged women who think they look wonderful but rarely do. Even leggings worn well are passé, to say the least - and date you more accurately than wrinkles could ever do. And the baggy sweater that usually tops them hides a good figure and simply makes an out-of-shape figure look even worse.

And you would never wear leggings with high-heeled shoes – would you?

A much better bet for everyday wear are chinos such as those Angela is wearing here. Team them with a shirt, a waistcoat and some canvas plimsolls or leather loafers for a much more up-to-date look. You could also try coloured jeans or a pair of brightly coloured capri pants.

DON'T BE A FASHION VICTIM

If you don't want to appear dated, you should certainly NOTICE what is going on in the world of fashion, and evolve your wardrobe so it is reasonably up-to-date. But one thing you should try to avoid is paying too much attention to the more wild flights of fancy of the fashion world – from street fashion that changes ten times a season, to couture. Don't feel obliged to be seen wearing the latest thing. If it is something that happens to suit you – fine but unless you're super-rich, be wary of buying something ultra-trendy now, because you won't get a lot of wear out of it before it has to be dumped.

Says Ceril, 'The best idea is to have a wardrobe based on fairly classic shapes and colours and add to it each season with one or two bigger fashion items and several up-to-the-minute inexpensive accessories, as long as they all suit you. It's quite easy to update a wardrobe with new season's colours and styles in t-shirts, jewellery, belt, bag and shoes.

'Look at the fashion magazines and style programmes; see what is in the shops and what people are wearing - and interpret the trends. Learn to pick up on what will look good on you and IGNORE what won't. Check out the new season's colours and if one of your less good colours is this year's Big Thing, keep it for small pieces or items away from your face and team with one of your better colours.'

DRESSING FOR YOUR AGE

Every woman has a fear of looking like 'mutton dressed as lamb'. To my mind, however, just as bad is the woman who insists upon wearing great–great–grannie clothes the moment she hits 50. With the help of Linda and Angela, who do some modelling, we examine this old chestnut of dressing for your age.

There is only a fine line between dressing to look younger, gracefully, and making an idiot of yourself with clothes that are far too young for you. But very few women do, in fact, opt for a young and girlish look. Most, fearing the 'mutton' tag more than anything, go the other way, and wear drab and mumsy clothes long before they need. (In fact, there is NEVER a need).

Here we run through some clothes considerations and point out mistakes you're likely to make, either way. The comments are only a guide – adapt them to suit your own personality, age, lifestyle, and so on.

Colours and materials

Too young: mixing lots of different brights; PVC, rubber, some leathers.
• **Too old:** all beige; dull grannie prints; all black; towelling (except for sport).

Skirt lengths and styles

Too young: extremely short; extremely tight.
Too old: mid-calf length; gathered; voluminous; tailored pleats.

Evening wear

Too young: strapless gowns exposing flabby arms/neck/back/etc (OK if you're very well-toned – check out back view!); too much cleavage showing; flounces and frills.
Too old: scarves used to cover the bits mentioned above – everyone knows that trick.

Casual

Too young: short shorts (unless your legs are perfect and you're on holiday); see-throughs (not wonderful on any age); going bare-legged with anything other than trousers or long skirts (unless your legs are perfect and/or you're on holiday).
Too old: shell suits *(you don't have one, do you?!)*; tweedy baggy country look (unless roaming your estate); twin-set and pearls; fussy printed polyester dresses.

Accessories

• **Too young:** very high heels; huge platforms; white shoes; baseball caps; Doc Marten/Caterpillar-type boots unless walking/gardening or similar (Timberlands are OK with a casual outfit); plastic anything.
Too old: frumpy shoes; slippers; head-scarves tied à la Queen of England.

Dressing too young

Angela models how not to do it. Her suit fails on several counts – the dress neckline is a bit too low; the skirt a bit too high and much too tight. The jacket is also too tight where it buttons. The lime colour, while very trendy at the time Angela modelled, is rendered 'over the top' by the addition of the fuchsia detail.

Getting it right
Angela can wear a short and fitted lime green suit – *here's how*. Attention to detail and simplicity makes all the difference.

Dressing too old

Believe it or not, this is Angela again, all dressed up for the office or a semi-formal lunch, or whatever – and making herself look 20 years older than she is! The drab colour of the blouse is completely wrong for Angela and boring with the suit. The suit skirt is very ageing, with its pleats and it's mid-calf length. The shape of the court shoes is way out-of-date, the complete outfit is shapeless and the ageing, harsh hairline and pearls finish the effect off.

Getting it right
It is possible to look neat and efficient and young, too! Here Angela wears a simple straight-skirted belted coat dress and some up-to-date shoes. A less severe hairstyle finishes the look very well.

Dressing too mumsy

Linda owns this dress but brought it along to our studio knowing it to be a terrible mistake! Avoid, at all costs, polyester printed dresses with self belts, pleats or gathers and ending at mid calf. Avoid loud prints and avoid sleeves that finish around the elbow. All will conspire to make you look like a fashion dinosaur and twice your age.

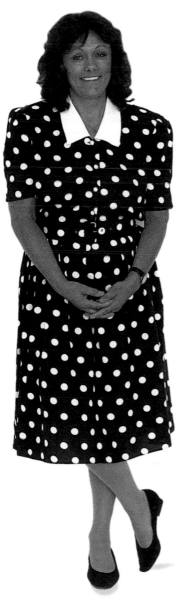

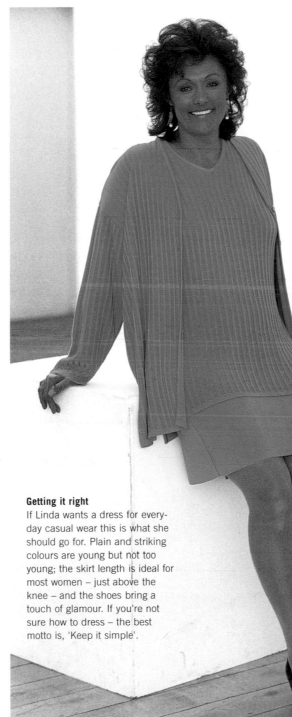

Getting it right
If Linda wants a dress for every-day casual wear this is what she should go for. Plain and striking colours are young but not too young; the skirt length is ideal for most women – just above the knee – and the shoes bring a touch of glamour. If you're not sure how to dress – the best motto is, 'Keep it simple'.

WARDROBE WORKOUT

Sue is a part-time GP and mother of two. Having paid little attention to her clothes since giving birth to her oldest daughter, now eight, Sue was desperate for some practical style suggestions. Sue, 39, had put on a stone since having children and, largely because of this surplus weight, hadn't bothered about her clothes for years. Her wardrobe was full of mumsy mid-length skirts and sensible jumpers and cardis – her typical wear for her 5-times-a-week surgery. Colours were dark to muted to white. Says Ceril, 'The outfit (left) is typical of the kind of thing Sue has been wearing for years. A safe and rather nondescript skirt with a knitted cardi that makes her look much larger than she really is (a neat size 10 in this photo). The skirt length, opaque tights and old-fashioned flattie shoes finish a dowdy image that does Sue no favours at all. 'Sue has chosen clothes that don't stand out – nothing to show off her figure.'

'But,' says Sue, 'I have little confidence in what to buy for myself now. I just know I need a new look, and I'd rather not spend too much money on any single item.'

'Sue is a "winter" person,' says Ceril. 'She is going to look really good in icy pastels, and in turquoisey blue and pinky or bluey reds. The muted, drab colours are making her "fade away". The colours I suggest will really bring her look alive and bring out her true personality.

'Sue has lost a stone in the 10 weeks, and also needs to rethink the shape of her clothes. She is quite small – at 5 foot 4 inches – and longer length and baggy skirts and fussy knits swamp her. She will suit above-the-knee straight skirts, and hip-length

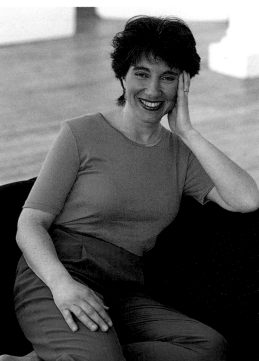

At home or for holidays, Sue really does suit these bright greens and blues in easy-care, easy-wear fabrics.

jackets, rather than the longer length she has preferred. Lighter shoes and tights – and a little make-up – will all help to lift her look.'

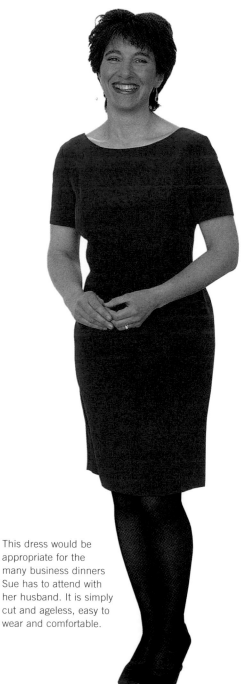

This dress would be appropriate for the many business dinners Sue has to attend with her husband. It is simply cut and ageless, easy to wear and comfortable.

Sue loved this suit, which is surprisingly inexpensive. If clothes are kept simple you can often get away with not spending a fortune. 'I am going to buy a couple of simple suits and wear them to work instead of my jumpers and skirts!' said Sue.

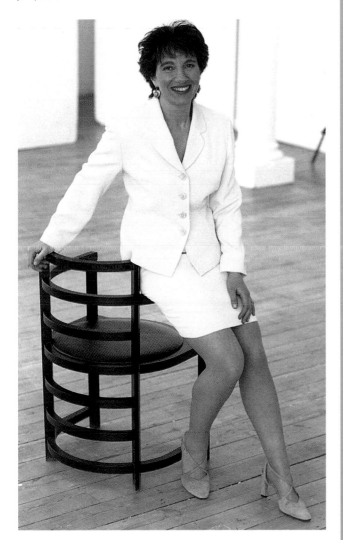

REVAMP YOUR WARDROBE

Now give your own wardrobe a workout. Allow as long as you can for each part of this exercise.

Part One

Go through absolutely everything in your current wardrobe, putting it all into one of four piles and remembering everything Ceril has taught you about style:

1 A pile of things you wear and that pass the style test.
2 A pile of things that you never wear and/or are doing you no favours. This pile you give away.
3 A pile of things that may have possibilities if you can find items to team with them.
4 And a pile of things that need mending/shortening/taking in or whatever.

Now do the same with your shoes, bags, belts, etc., teaming accessories up with suitable outfits from pile 1 and throwing out everything that really isn't going to be worn any more.
Now spot the gaps in your wardrobe (bearing in mind your own lifestyle) by checking down this capsule list of items that will be most useful:

● At least two or three good, classic things (e.g. suits, trouser suit, dress and jacket combinations) that you can wear frequently and maybe use the jackets or trousers or skirts with other items.
● Several bolder, smaller items to enliven the classics – shirts, waistcoats, bodies, sweaters, tunics.
● Several casual mix and matches for everyday wear – chinos, capris, jeans, with teaming tops.
● One or two outfits suitable for evening - separates allow more flexibility.
● Accessories to match all these outfits.

Now write a list of what sort of things you need to fill the gaps. If you've lost a lot of weight and/or haven't bought for ages, the gaps may be quite big but you can always build up a new wardrobe slowly over a period of time or maybe even check out one of the many excellent used-clothes stores for low-cost quality items.
Don't be afraid to buy a few inexpensive little high-fashion items – T-shirts in this season's colour, for instance, which will update and enliven your wardrobe considerably.

Part Two

Again allow as long as you can for this exercise, which is a shopping trip!
Now it's time to go and try on as many things as you can (preferably alone . . . your own judgement is something you need to learn to trust) in as many shops as you can. (*Take spare shoes, tights and T-shirt with you if intending to try various styles - the wrong accessories with an outfit can distract you from the right decision.*) A big department store with lots of concession shops within it is an excellent idea. Try, try, try. If an item passes the six-point checklist here, consider adding it to your wardrobe:

● Does it fit?
● Does the colour suit you?
● Does the style suit you?
● Does it go with other things in your wardrobe?
● Will you get plenty of usage out of it?
● Do you really like it?

*F*ew women – even most of the supermodels – have perfect figures.
In this workshop, Ceril Campbell makes the most of a variety of figure
shapes – and shows you what to avoid.

WORKSHOP 10 STYLE ASSESSMENT 2
DRESSING FOR YOUR SHAPE

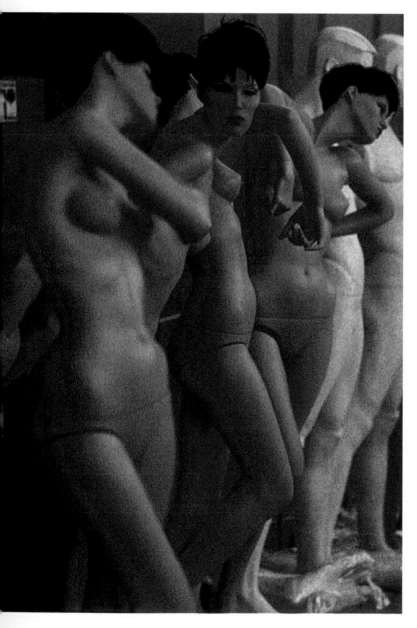

By the time we reach the 30s and 40s, most of us know only too well which bits of our bodies we dislike. Even with careful diet and plenty of toning exercise, basic body shape is something you have to live with. But, with the clever use of clothes – and that includes design, colour, material, length, and so on – to draw attention AWAY from your worst bits and TOWARDS your good points, you can make yourself look 100 per cent better proportioned.

Incredible, then, that very many of us actually do the reverse – we often choose clothes that make us look WORSE than we really are. So next time you go shopping – take a few minutes to look hard at each outfit you try on and ask yourself – is it REALLY doing your body any favours . . . or could you do better?

Over the next few pages, we use some of our 10-week participants as models. We persuaded them to wear outfits that didn't suit their figures at all (often things they had bought themselves) and tell you why. Then we put them into something much more flattering and again tell you why. Using these examples, plus the extra tips you'll find on each page, you'll find it hard to make those same mistakes again.

We hope you'll be inspired to go through your wardrobe and throw out those clothes that are doing your body no favours, right away!

HILARY
- minimizing hips and thighs

Hilary has an excellent figure
but, partly because her bust is quite small,
she tends to look 'hippy' in some outfits,
and her thighs are quite heavy compared
with her upper body.

If you're pear-shaped:

DO
• Wear small shoulder pads to balance out your body.
• Wear darker colours on the bottom half.
• Wear plain colours on the bottom half.
• Wear vertical seams or stripes on bottom half.
• Wear shaped, not straight-cut long-line jackets to cover hips and thighs.
• Wear tapered, slim-legged trousers (but skimming over thighs).

DON'T
• Wear bulky fabrics on your bottom half.
• Wear tops that finish on the widest part of your hips/thighs.
• Wear belts too tight around the waist; this will make hips look bigger.

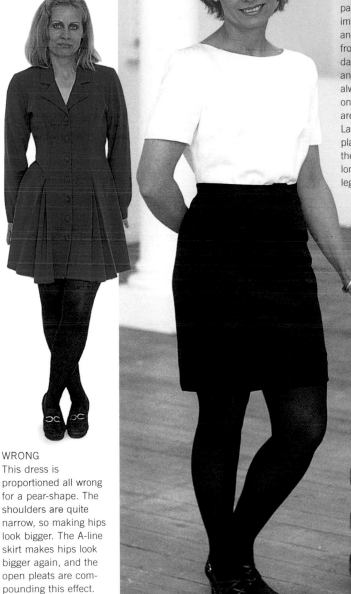

WRONG
This dress is proportioned all wrong for a pear-shape. The shoulders are quite narrow, so making hips look bigger. The A-line skirt makes hips look bigger again, and the open pleats are compounding this effect.

What a difference! This dress has plenty of plus-points for Hilary. The wide neckline and lightly padded shoulders are creating a wide shoulder line to balance her silhouette. The pale top is increasing the impact of the bust and arms and draws attention away from the lower body, and the dark skirt diminishes the hips and thighs – dark colours always diminish and light ones always make what they are covering seem larger. Lastly, the dark tights and plain court shoes to match the skirt help to create a longer, leaner line to Hilary's legs. Lovely!

PAMELA
- a typical apple

Pamela, like many women
in their late 40s, 50s and 60s,
is an 'apple'; with a large waist
and tummy, and slim
arms and legs.

When this photo was taken,
Pam had already lost over
3 inches from around her
waist – but this shirtwaister
dress (her own) adds more
inches than she'd taken off!
It's also the kind of
'grannie' dress that no
woman of any age should
consider going near! The
print is unflattering; the bit
of dark belt showing draws
attention to the stomach;
the slightly blouson-top
adds inches at each side of
her waist and the pleats
hanging straight from the
waist make her look wide
all the way down. The
dowdy length skirt finishes
the (unflattering) picture.

Apple shapes should aim to skim
over their middles with well-cut
clothes that give long, clean
unfussy lines. This tweed trouser
suit makes Pam look a stone lighter
– and 20 years younger. Neutral
colours can be very glamorous if
they are worn in the right way, and
there is no need to discount wearing a trouser suit whatever your
age. If your apple shape means
that you find the waistband tight,
go for suits with some Lycra or
stretch in the waistband - there are
plenty around. The silk T-shirt top
worn over the trousers is a better
bet for apples than a top tucked in;
and the slim legs and arms of this
suit add to the slim lines.

If you're apple-shaped:

DO:
• Keep detail round the
waist to a minimum.
• Create slightly angular
lines to your outline with
light shoulder pads or
tailored shoulders; edge-
to-edge jackets and
straight skirts or straight-
legged trousers.
• Wear tunic-style tops
over trousers and skirts,
rather than tuck them in.
• Wear short skirts to show
off slim legs.

DON'T:
• Choose loose-pleated
skirts; pick stitched pleats
instead.
• Choose gathered skirts.
• Wear pockets anywhere
near the waistline.
• Choose jodhpurs if you
have thin legs and a big
stomach.
• Choose wide-legged
floating trousers.
• Choose formal suits with
waist-length or cropped
jackets.

KAY
- coping with a big bust

Kay has a 39-inch bust which can seem even bigger because the rest of her is relatively slim. She doesn't like her bust and tries to disguise it with big baggy tops and blouses. A tailored look is a better approach.

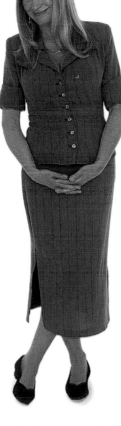

If you like your big bust and want to show it off, this could be a good outfit, but for Kay, it isn't. It accentuates her top-heavy shape because the jacket is too tight and is straining at the buttons; there is a horizontal seam across the bustline, drawing attention to it. The sleeves finish at the lower edge of the bust, drawing attention to that area, and the waisted jacket also makes the bust more obvious. The long-length skirt also covers up the asset that Kay should be using to detract attention from her top half – those long, long legs!

Kay couldn't have done better if this suit had been specially designed for her. The dark navy, well-cut jacket skims over her bustline and the self-coloured chemise underneath creates a simple, understated line to the whole upper body area. The eye is drawn to the pale short skirt and to the legs – exactly the effect we wanted to achieve.

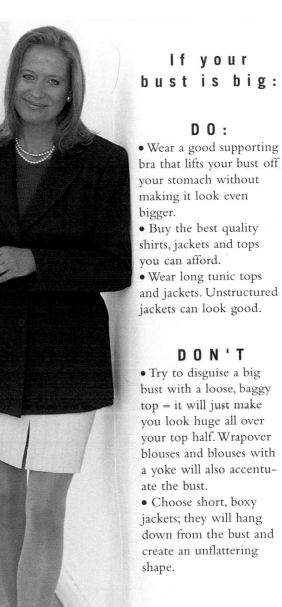

If your bust is big:

DO:
• Wear a good supporting bra that lifts your bust off your stomach without making it look even bigger.
• Buy the best quality shirts, jackets and tops you can afford.
• Wear long tunic tops and jackets. Unstructured jackets can look good.

DON'T
• Try to disguise a big bust with a loose, baggy top – it will just make you look huge all over your top half. Wrapover blouses and blouses with a yoke will also accentuate the bust.
• Choose short, boxy jackets; they will hang down from the bust and create an unflattering shape.

Short-cuts for Sally

Sal has a nice curvy figure, but she wants advice on dressing for those curves and wants to look taller – she's 5 foot 3 inches, with quite a short body.

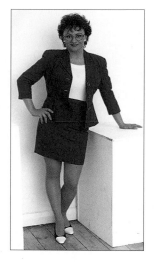

Sal wears a lot of black, and thought this suit would look good on her – but it's a disaster! The short jacket is cutting her body in two and making it look too 'boxy'. Sal has a good waist and the boxy cut loses it. The double breast and heavy lapel detail is also doing nothing for her bustline, making her look bulky. The wide sleeves are swamping Sal and adding width, too. The short skirt forms another box shape, compounding the problem. The shoulders are too heavy and wide for Sal and the polo neck accentuates Sal's short neck.

Here's a similar TYPE of suit that works so much better. Here's why. It's all one colour – if you take one colour through an outfit, it will always make you look taller and slimmer. The jacket suit Sal's curves, and is a slightly longer length and single-breasted, slimming down all of Sal's upper body, particularly her bust. The narrow sleeves suit Sal much better, and the little white low-necked body elongates her neck and diminishes her jaw-line. Isn't it amazing how two outfits so similar in intention can produce two such contrasting images?

If you're a bit short and curvy:

DO:
- Go for one main colour from top to toe; with tights and shoes that match each other, too.
- Go for slim skirts and fitted jackets which follow your curves.
- Wear slim trousers and mid-heeled shoes.

DON'T:
- Wear voluminous clothes; they will swamp you.
- Wear large patterns; they will have the same effect
- Wear long skirts.
- Wear very high heels – they will simply help to make you look out of proportion.

Downsizing Linda

Linda has lost well over a stone
on our ten-week programme,
but still has some to lose. She
wants advice for dressing slim
in the meantime!

This really is a dress out of
Linda's wardrobe - but she
admits it's not her style! Linda
is a size 16-18, with big bust,
waist, hips and thighs. This
dress is managing to get it
all wrong for someone of
Linda's size. It has an
unflattering neckline and the
cutaway sleeves are not good
if your upper arms are a bit
flabby (something that can
happen over 40, however slim
you are). The white belt draws
attention to the waist and
tummy area and also to a
droopy bust (Linda needs a
better bra). The lightly gathered skirt again makes her
midriff look larger than it is –
and those bright horizontal
stripes are a no-no for any
body area you want to slim
down. Oh, yes – and the length
of the dress is decidedly
mumsy and hides Linda's slim
calves. WHOEVER designed
this dress?

And whoever said larger women can't wear
fitted clothes? Linda looks TWO stones lighter than
in her 'before' picture, with this terrific ensemble of
black crew-neck fine-knit jumper, single-breasted
jacket in fine black stripes on pale beige, and stretch
jodhpurs to match, all finished with a pair of black
jodhpur boots.
This is the exception that proves the rule – although
we've said that pale colours enlarge and dark ones
diminish, in this instance the pale beige doesn't have
that effect as Linda's colouring really suits paler colours
– the dark buttons draw the eye to the centre; the
jacket is very well cut and neatly covers Linda's 'butt',
and the jodhpurs show off her slim calves and ankles.

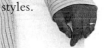

If you're plump:

DO:
• Go for plain materials
rather than wild patterns.
• Choose vertical stripes.
• Choose fine materials
rather than thick ones –
e.g. thin knits, not
chunky ones; silk, not
satin; linen, not cotton
towelling, and so on.
• Go for casually tailored
styles.

DON'T:
• Choose long flowing
garments in bold patterns.
• Choose shiny fabrics.
• Choose clothes that are
too tight.
• Choose puff sleeves or
anything 'girlie'.

Short-waisted Sue

Sue has a lovely neat figure, but quite a short waist. When we first met her she was wearing almost everything that is exactly wrong for a short waist – especially if, like Sue, you aren't very tall.

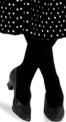

Starting from the top: the blouse is too wide and unstructured, making Sue look bulky around the waist. The sleeves finish at exactly the wrong point – right on the waist. The wide bright belt draws attention to the waist and shortens it further. The gathered skirt materializing from under the belt adds another bulky layer. For a taller women, the skirt length would not be too bad, but Sue is swamped, and the shoes which don't match the tights shorten the overall look too.

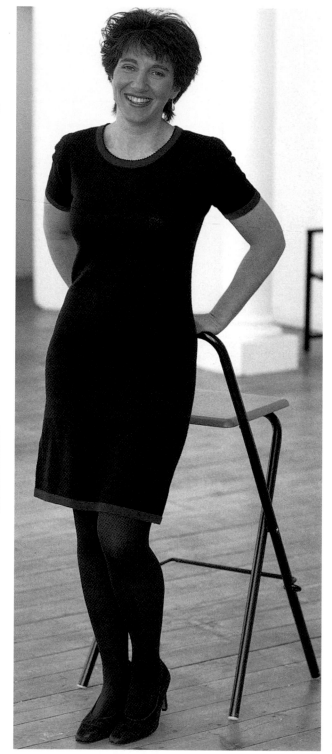

If you're petite and short-waisted:

DO:
• Wear shift dresses.
• Wear single breasted jackets to hip length (no longer).
• Wear empire line or drop waist dresses.
• Keep lines simple.
• Wear tunic tops with long narrow trousers.

DON'T:
• Wear blouses and skirts, for choice.
• Wear wide stiff belts – a narrow, fluid hipster belt is a good choice if you have to belt up.
• Ever wear gathered skirts or blouses with no darts (unless worn outside trousers or skirts).
• Wear fussy clothes.

Although navy isn't one of Sue's own best colours, it does suit most women – if this dark navy isn't perfect, then a lighter French navy would be an alternative. This plain and simple dress lets Sue's figure speak for itself. It skims over her waist, creating a long, lean line. The length is much better for her, and the lowish rounded neckline draws attention to that area rather than the waist. The master touch of red trimming at neck and hem takes the eye up, then down. It never lingers around the middle, as it did all too long on Sue's 'before' outfit.

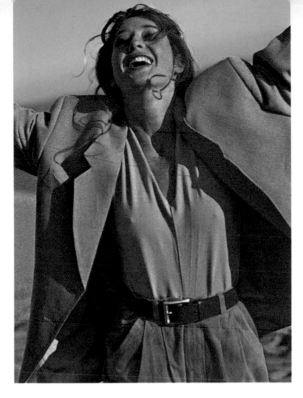

ENERGY SOURCES

The Vital You

Energy. . . vitality. . . sparkle. . . the missing ingredients in so many women's lives. And yet an abundance of energy, both mental and physical, IS the master key to a fulfilling life because it has a profound effect upon what you do, how you feel and how you look. Think back to ten or twenty years ago when it was normal for you to wake up refreshed and alert, keen to get up and on with the day; when you looked forward to what lay ahead; felt excited by challenges, and packed more into a day than you sometimes do now in a week.

Now your 'norm' is to wake up reluctantly and wish you could spend the day in bed with the phone off the hook – even a good book is too much effort to read. If only you could get back that youthful *joie de vivre*; if only you could look in the mirror and see bright-eyed enthusiasm. But, sadly, loss of vitality is just part of getting older, isn't it? You slow down, lose your edge.

There are two keys to getting your vitality back. The first is in embracing the energy-givers. From what you eat to how you breathe, from learning to relax to planning your days better and getting your body fit to cope – you need to use the energy-givers to empower you.

The second is in clearing your life of the energy-sappers – the physical and emotional factors that are bringing you down. Minor ailments, boredom, poor sleep patterns, overwork and poor nutrition are just a few of the energy-sappers that many of us live with every day. This second section of the book aims to help you do both. The real, pure feeling of zest for life – of feeling in control again – is something you can't fake, but when you've got it, is guaranteed to melt the years away.

I f you lack energy, the first thing you need to do is check out your general health, because many physical problems can deplete energy (if only because 'it's one more thing to worry about').

WORKSHOP **11** HEALTH CHECK

Go through the health checklist opposite and every time you tick a symptom, refer to the Action column for what to do. Many of the symptoms are covered in other workshops to which you'll be guided; for others you'll find recommended courses of action, or you will be asked to see your appropriate practitioner. Don't ignore symptoms that need a professional check-up! For example, 10% of cases of unexplained constant tiredness are due to an illness that has gone undetected, such as thyroid problems, rheumatics or fibromyalgia, anaemia or diabetes. After all, you do value your own body more than you value your car — don't you?

Eight simple ways to a healthier you

❶ Regular all-over check ups, e.g. Well Woman clinic

❷ Quit smoking

❸ Moderate your alcohol consumption

❹ Sleep, rest and relaxation

❺ Fresh air

❻ Regular exercise

❼ Healthy diet, healthy weight

❽ Enjoy life

Health Checklist

Tick which symptoms relate to you under every section:

Symptom	Action
Stress-related Symptoms	
❏ Disrupted eating patterns	Workshop 13 (even if you need to slim)
❏ Digestive problems	Ditto
❏ Insomnia	Workshops 15, 16, 17
❏ Tiredness not linked to insomnia	Workshops 13 - 15 and 17 - 24 plus see GP
❏ Unexplained minor aches and pains	Check again at end of 10-week programme If not gone, see GP
❏ Recurrent minor infections	Ditto
❏ Palpitations/breathlessness	See GP. If cleared, Workshops 14 and 15 will help
❏ Depression/crying/fear/panic	See GP or counsellor; Workshops 14-24
❏ Irritability/aggression	Ditto
❏ Lack of concentration/memory	Workshops 14,15,16
❏ Loss of interest in sex/social life	Workshops 21,22, also see GP, also refer to sex symptom section below
Sex symptoms	
❏ Pre-menstrual syndrome	Workshop 13, see GP, regular exercise, natural diuretics – *e.g. celery, fennel, lettuce, melon, citrus, tomatoes, parsley*
❏ Heavy/prolonged/frequent/ painful periods	See GP; consider hormone treatment
❏ Painful intercourse	Consider hormone treatment; try lubricant; see Workshop 21
❏ Lack of sex drive	Workshops 12, 13, 14, 15, 16, 21, 22, 24. See GP/counsellor at end of 10 weeks if no improvement
Aches and pains	
❏ Back/neck pain	See GP, also Workshops 3, 4, see osteopath, check chairs, bed, driving position
❏ Headaches	See GP; Workshops 13, 15, see optician
❏ Rheumatic pain	See GP; homeopathy, herbalism, Workshop 13
❏ Joint pain	See GP for suitable treatment, exercise and diet; also Workshop 4.
❏ Toothache	See dentist
Frequent minor illnesses	
❏ Colds	Workshops 13, 14, extra vitamin C and zinc, Workshops 15 and 24
❏ Sore throat	See GP; consider stress levels
❏ Gum problems	See dentist; extra vitamin C, careful mouth hygiene, daily flossing
❏ Sore/red eyes	See GP; extra vitamin C, consider allergy
❏ Hair loss	See GP, check stress levels
❏ Bronchitis	Workshops 3, 4, 13, 14 , see GP
❏ Irregular bowel movements	Workshops 13, 14, 15, see GP
❏ Poor digestion	Ditto
❏ Thrush	Twice daily bio yoghurt, pro-bacteria, proprietary cream from pharmacy
❏ Cystitis	See GP; plenty of water to drink
Menopause plus	
❏ Hot flushes	See GP, consider hormone treatment, vitamin E supplements and evening primrose oil
❏ Sleeplessness	Workshops 14, 15, 16
❏ Lack of sex drive	See sex symptom section above
❏ Fatigue	Workshops 12-16 and all of Section 3
❏ Weight gain	Workshop 2, then 13
❏ Stress incontinence	See GP; pelvic floor exercise

Ten symptoms you should never ignore

❶ Chest pains on exertion

❷ Unexplained weight loss or gain

❸ Unexplained pain anywhere in body lasting more than a few days

❹ Unexplained fatigue continuing for more than a week or so after trying all remedies suggested above

❺ Skin changes

❻ Internal bleeding other than menstruation

❼ Breast lumps

❽ Continuing headache

❾ Unexplained fainting/dizziness

❿ Nausea/sickness lasting more than a day or two

*M*ost of us underestimate the importance of clever and thoughtful management of our own time. Yet with streamlining strategies and sensible planning and control, the extra time you buy yourself can make all the difference to your energy levels and your life.

WORKSHOP 12 TIME MANAGEMENT

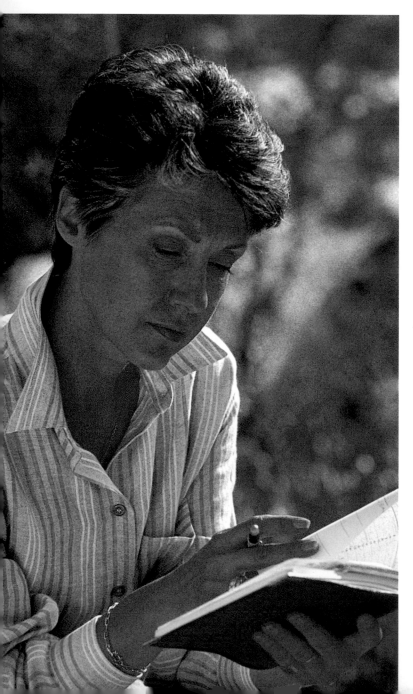

We all waste time, even when we think we don't, and cutting down that wastage is vital for women who, it is acknowledged, generally have to pack more into their days than the average man – 'doing it all', rather than 'having it all'. I hardly know one woman for whom 'finding time' ISN'T a never-ending problem.

The 'busy busy syndrome', with life always half an hour behind schedule; with long, long hours and never any time for YOU means that you are living in a permanently stressful, energy-draining environment. Buying extra time with some simple strategies means that stress levels reduce, energy increases – and you're on the way to getting the life you want.

Your Time Diary

First, keep your own 'time diary' for three days.

● Make three columns – 1. *time*, – 2. *what you did*, and leave the third column blank for now.

● List everything you do from the time you wake to going to sleep. Obviously, keeping the diary is going to take up some of your precious time but it will be time well spent in this instance!

● Now carry on with the workshop and fill in the blank column afterwards.

Monday 7.15 am
7.35 am
8.00 am

Planning Ahead

It is hard to manage time efficiently without lists. If you already live by lists, make sure yours really work for you.

You need a 'to do today' list – ideally broken up into professional life and personal life. And you need a 'to do this week' list. I also like a 'long-term' list, but that's optional.

Write your 'today' list the night before (it will help you sleep well). In the morning go through your today list and ruthlessly cross out anything that isn't really necessary and/or that you don't really want to do. For this, you need to get into the habit of being firm (see right). Also, Parkinson's law dictates that a job will expand to fill the time you have for it, so rather than have this happen to you, nominate how much time each item on your list should take, and try to stick to it.

Every day, work through your today list from the top. Aim to get through the list in all but the most unexpected circumstances. At the end of the day, make the list for the following day, with anything that didn't do that day at the top. If, after two weeks, an item is still on the list and still not done, either do it immediately, or take it off the list and forget it.

Two other kinds of lists it is worth making:

TV LIST – at the weekend, go through the viewing for the week ahead and make a note of anything you really want to watch (ask your self *why* you want to watch it) and don't watch anything else; and a MENU LIST – particularly if you have to cook for people other than yourself. Always plan meals on a weekly basis and shop after you've planned what you will eat. This will save panic trips to the supermarket every other day, it will save time and your energy by having another area of your life settled in advance. It will also save money.

Be Firm

Being firm, both with others and yourself, is perhaps the biggest time-saver of all.

- Where possible, never do overtime you aren't being paid for or don't want to do. If beginning a new job, start with this firmly in mind as it is harder to refuse once you've already set a precedent.
- Accept that it is better to finish a task competently than to take twice as long to do it perfectly. Anyway, perfectionism isn't admired by others, It Is disliked because it makes everyone else feel guilty.
- Keep meetings as short as possible by keeping focused on the subject and if colleagues stray off the point, firmly bring them back.
- Delegate (see also overleaf).

In Your Personal Life

- Never agree to do anything you don't want to do. Sounds simple, but we almost all do accept invitations we'd rather refuse, agree to charitable works we don't have time for, let people invite themselves for the weekend even though we don't get along with them all that well. . . *you know the score.* You do it because you want to be liked. But there are better ways to be liked and most of these demands on your time are cup-board love and no more. Are the people making demands the people you want to be liked by, anyway? And isn't it better to like yourself, first? Say 'no' and start practising now. Say 'no' anyway you like – directly, diplomatically, with a white lie. But say no.
- Learn to know your limitations – keep your commitments within the bounds of what you can do without exhausting yourself. There is no need to feel guilty for this; it is common sense.

Be Fit

Physical fitness helps you to get through almost everything in your life more quickly and more efficiently. This is because being fit means being stronger (so chores are got through more easily); being fit means a better supply of oxygen to your brain (so you have better mental alertness to do mental tasks, can read quicker, absorb information quicker, and so on). Being fit also means less chance of being laid up in bed with illness.

So check out the Stamina workshop and make sure to use some of the time you save in other ways, by keeping yourself as fit as possible.

Woke up. Listened to news on TV. Got up and got ready. Left home for work (no time for breakfast . . .)

Could have got ready while listening to news then had time for breakfast.

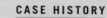
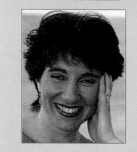
Take a Look at Your Sleeping Patterns

Getting enough good-quality sleep is vital, which is why a whole workshop is devoted to just that (see Workshop 15). However, one in three of us stay in bed longer than we need. Too much sleep is not necessary, and many people can cut down the time they spend in bed by up to an hour with no ill effects and the benefit of an extra seven hours a week of time. So try these tips for saving sleep time:

● Don't go to bed until you are tired.

● Leave a window open and never have heating on in the bedroom while you sleep. Using these strategies you are likely to wake up slightly earlier than usual and feel more refreshed, avoiding the temptation of having a 'lie in'.

● Get up as soon as you wake up; don't linger.

● Set the alarm to wake you 30 minutes earlier than usual for a week. See if you notice any difference in how you feel during the day. If you don't feel any worse, take another half hour off the following week. You may even feel better – time in bed that you don't need increases sluggishness.

Be Aware of Time

It is perfectly OK sometimes to do absolutely nothing, as you will find out in Workshop 15. You want to set aside that time on a regular basis and enjoy it; let it revive you. It is also fine to daydream if it helps you to plan out what you really want and plot your future. But don't fritter away time – or allow other people to fritter away time for you.

Here are some examples of good time frittered, not spent:

● Watching TV just because it is on. If you can, move to another room or turn it off. If not, wear earplugs and read or write or work on a hobby, or anything on your list (see previous page).

● Listening to gossip or similar. Be polite if you meet people you know in the street or in a shop or so forth but don't feel obliged to stand and chat for ages if you are busy. Be firm, move on.

● Reading gossip or similar. Don't buy trash papers that offer little except show-biz gossip and voyeurism on other people's lives. A good book will teach you more about human nature. Talking of books – NEVER carry on reading a book if, after ten pages, you find it boring. If you want to know the ending – read the last few pages.

● Listening to door-to-door callers. If a salesman or missionary arrives at your door, never encourage him or her; say straightaway 'no thank you', say good day and shut the door.

● People or things keeping you waiting. It's surprising how often you find yourself 'hanging around' for ten minutes or so just waiting. Don't waste it, use it. Say, you've cooked a supper for friends and everything is ready but they are late arriving. Don't stand in the kitchen checking your watch. Do a 10-minute task on your list or read a few pages of your book. While a pan of water comes to the boil for the pasta, tidy out the fridge, or ring a friend. Never go to an appointment or meeting without something to do in the event of being kept waiting.

Delegate

Women are often quite poor at delegating, especially at home. But if you live with a partner and/or children over the age of five, they can and should all help out. After all, if you have, say, three other people in the household and each of them spends 20 minutes a day doing chores you used to do, that's a whole hour of your time saved. And, as research shows that the average woman spends SIX hours a day on home-related tasks, including shopping and cooking, you need to save as much time as you can! If you have spent years NOT delegating, this new tough line may take a while - and some determination - to bring about. But stand firm! It can be done.

Here is the route to follow:

1 Explain to them why it is that they should become more involved in the routine of the home.

2 Explain what it is they should start doing (e.g. small children tidying their rooms, older children doing the dishes, partner ironing own clothes).

3 Remind them now and then.

4 Don't do it yourself.

5 If all else fails, employ paid help and explain to the reluctant helpers that you can no longer afford the designer clothes/fine wine holidays/expensive presents they have come to expect because the cash has had to be diverted. If you already have paid help, remember to let her/him do the work rather than sit at the table drinking coffee and eating biscuits and watching you do it.

Learn Time-saving Strategies

Sometimes you'll be doing things the same old way out of habit. But a few new tricks will save you time. Here are a few suggestions; think up some more of your own:

• Beating a trail round the shops for anything from clothes to presents is a waste of time and energy when virtually anything you want can be bought by telephone, fax, computer, the Internet or mail order and sent virtually anywhere. If you pay by credit card you are protected.

• Pay all regular bills on direct debit.

• Never cook an evening meal without making double quantities for the freezer.

• Dress using one colour as your signature colour. This saves having to spend ages trying to co-ordinate everything, and saves time on deciding what to pack for holidays.

• Have an easy-care hairstyle.

• Double up as much as you can; e.g., don't JUST see a friend – see a friend *and* go to the art exhibition you have been trying to get to for ages.

ANALYSING YOUR TIME DIARY

Right. Now go back through your own time diary bearing in mind the above tips, and see what time you could have saved.

• How many things did you do that you should have delegated?

• How many things did you do that you didn't really want to do?

• How much time did you allow to be frittered? And so on.

Write your comments in blank column three and then roughly estimate how much time you could have saved each day. Vow to get in the habit of being time- efficient in future. That doesn't mean you need to lead a regimented life with no fun – far from it. Saving time on things that don't matter means you will have more time for what you really want to do. Write a list of all those things (anything from seeing more of your friends and relatives to travelling – Section Three will give you many more ideas), pin it up somewhere you see every day and do it.

To Sum Up:

To save time you must:

• Be firm with yourself and with others.

• Not drift – be aware of the time you are using, and why.

• Plan ahead.

• Take new time-saving ideas on board.

• Delegate, delegate, delegate.

• Be fit and be disciplined about sleep.

• Keep your commitments within the bounds of what you can do without exhausting yourself.

J ust as a car needs the right fuel to run efficiently and perform well, so does your body. The well-fed body is less likely to suffer from mental or physical sluggishness; from tiredness, minor ailments, colds and a general feeling of being 'under par'. Sound eating geared to your own needs can also help your body cope better with the pressures, pace and pollutants of modern life. So begin thinking of food as fuel to empower you and enhance your performance, and you will see just how important it is to eat right for energy.

WORKSHOP 13 EATING FOR ENERGY

The Energy Enhancers

So what IS the best possible fuel for your body? You need to eat healthily, that's for sure – a varied diet containing all the vital nutrients in the right proportions, as outlined by the World Health Organisation. This means getting plenty of carbohydrate foods (such as potatoes, grains, pulses), enough protein foods (such as lean meat, poultry, fish, dairy and vegetable proteins) and a little fat, preferably from fish, vegetable and seed oils. It means plenty of fruit and vegetables. And it means cutting back on the foods that upset this balance – going easy on the chocolate, the chips, the gâteaux, pastries and cream, for instance.

In the quest for feeling great, however, we can take it further than that. Some nutrients are particularly important in maintaining energy levels, and so foods that contain high levels of those nutrients can be aptly called the 'superfoods' – and a diet rich in the superfoods will indeed be five-star fuel. What you need to do is incorporate as many of these energy-enhancing foods into your generally healthy diet as you possibly can.

Let's look at these 'energy enhancers' in detail.

Magnesium. A deficiency of magnesium is linked to chronic fatigue syndrome, ME, low energy levels and fluctuating blood sugar levels.

Zinc and Iron. Both vital for maintaining energy levels and healthy red blood cells, especially if you are exercising more or if you have heavy periods.

Vitamins E and the B group. Essential for making and keeping healthy red blood cells.

The antioxidants - the vitamin A precursor, beta-carotene, vitamins C and E, and the mineral selenium. The antioxidants neutralize the effect of the 'free radicals' in our bodies which cause cell and tissue damage and are the most likely cause of the ageing process and several of the degenerative diseases, such as Alzheimer's, heart disease and some cancers. The antioxidants are also vital in fighting the pollutants of modern life, such as pesticides and other chemicals in the food chain, and radiation. Garlic is also considered to be a powerful antioxidant.

An energy-enhancing diet will not only be high in the nutrients and foods we've discussed above but will also be low in those that have a negative effect on your energy or are of little or no nutritional value. These are:

Alcohol. A glass of wine with your evening meal, preferably organic wine, is fine. A little alcohol can be good for your heart, literally, and good for your soul. But more than a little is not a good idea. Drinking too much alcohol robs your body of the vitamin B group and vitamin C which as we've seen are vital for your health and energy. Also, because alcohol is akin to refined sugar, it will send your blood sugar levels soaring then dipping out of control, especially if you drink without eating. Result? You feel tired and terrible.

Sugar. The myth is that we need sugar for energy (glucose, too, an even more easily absorbed form of sugar) but we don't. A snack or drink high in sugar – a simple carbohydrate – and low in other nutrients will send your blood sugar crazy just like alcohol does. It works as a very short-term boost but unless you eat something nutritious shortly after, you will soon feel less energetic/more fatigued than before. The best foods for long-term energy are the ones that ensure a steady blood sugar level, such as wholegrains, fresh vegetables and lean proteins. White sugar is also the only food that is completely nutrient-deficient apart from the calories it contains.

Junk foods. If your diet is high in commercially produced sugary and/or fatty snacks and meals – like cakes, biscuits, pies, takeaways, chocolate, desserts and sweets – your body will suffer in two ways. Either you will not be eating enough of the nutrient-rich, energy-enhancing, healthy foods as discussed earlier

The Energy Robbers

(something's got to go!), or you will be eating both, and almost inevitably eating too many calories and you will end up overweight. Overweight in itself is an energy-robber. Carrying more than a few pounds of surplus fat is, if you don't already know, exhausting.

Caffeine. Thought of as a 'pick-me-up' and a stimulant, unfortunately caffeine also appears to produce its own 'low' in your body after the 'high'. In other words if you use coffee, tea, chocolate, cola or other caffeine-containing foods and drinks to boost your energy, you will later probably suffer a rebound effect and feel worse than before. Look to more caffeine to help you feel better, and that downward spiral is on its way.

Where to find the energy boosters

Beta-carotene:
orange, yellow and dark green vegetables, especially carrots, sweet potatoes, pumpkin and squash, tomatoes, spinach, broccoli, watercress, sweetcorn; orange fruits such as cantaloupe melon, mangoes, apricots and peaches

Vitamin B¹ (*thiamine*):
sunflower seeds, brown rice, wholegrain cereals, yeast extract, wheatgerm, pulses, brazil nuts, sprouting seeds, other nuts and seeds

Vitamin B² (*riboflavin*):
yeast extract, almonds, wheatgerm, cheese, mushrooms, broccoli, yoghurt, pulses, other nuts, eggs

Vitamin B³ (*niacin*):
yeast extract, pulses, whole wheat, brown rice, barley, eggs, meat and fish

Vitamin B⁶ (*pyridoxine*):
wheatgerm, soya, oats, walnuts, other nuts and pulses, bananas, avocados, wholegrains, meat, fish, green vegetables, sweet potatoes

Vitamin B¹²:
egg yolk, cheese, yeast extract, milk, fortified soya milk, seaweed

Vitamin C (*ascorbic acid*):
red peppers and chillies, blackcurrants, parsley, oranges, and all other fresh fruit and vegetables. (*Heat and light destroy vitamin, so fruits and vegetables must be stored in cool dark conditions and eaten as soon after purchase as possible; raw or lightly cooked.*)

Vitamin E (*tocopherol*):
sunflower oil, other pure vegetable oils, nuts, seeds, sweet potatoes, avocados, asparagus, green vegetables, barley, soya beans, brown rice

Iron:
meat, wholegrains, eggs, dark leafy greens, pulses, nuts and seeds, wheatgerm, dried apricots and peaches

Magnesium:
green vegetables, other vegetables, nuts, seeds, pulses, meat, fish and seafood, figs, bananas, brown rice

Zinc:
meat, wholegrains, fish and seafood, eggs, nuts and pulses

Selenium:
liver, kidneys, lean meat, fish and seafood, wholegrains

ソffffff

A high caffeine intake also depletes the body's minerals, including magnesium and zinc – another important reason to keep intake low.

Chemicals in food. Pesticides and other chemicals used for mass production of food can deplete or destroy the vital elements in the earth, such as magnesium and selenium, which is likely already to be depleted due to over-farming. Chemicals will also remain in and on our food, giving the antioxidants even harder work to do. Antibiotic residues in meat and dairy products may disrupt our immune systems. The answer? Choose organic food grown or produced whenever possible by people you know (grown by you, even better).

Allergens. Approximately one in 10 people suffer from some form of food allergy which can easily deplete energy. A wide variety of foods can produce allergic reactions, but the most common ones are wheat-based products, dairy produce, particularly cow's milk and cheese, berries and eggs. Food allergies can cause stomach bloating, lethargy, skin problems and headache. If you think you may have an allergy it is wise to see a practitioner who can arrange testing. If you want to self-test, cut out one food at a time from your diet for a period of 2 weeks each and if your symptoms disappear you may be allergic to that food. If on eating the food again the symptoms re-appear that food is probably the cause. Substitute rye or other grain breads for wheat bread, rice cakes or rye crackers for wheat crackers, and soya milk or goats' milk and cheese for cows' milk and cheese. As you are unlikely to be allergic to more than one or two foods, avoiding these foods won't harm the nutritional balance of your diet.

Crash dieting. A diet very low in calories causes extra free radicals to roam the body and destroy healthy cells – aggravated by the fact that most crash diets are woefully short in antioxidants. Crash diets also cause fatigue and loss of lean body tissue (muscle), essential for a healthy metabolic rate, strength and energy.

Two other factors can affect your body's absorption of the nutrients you need for energy:

Smoking
depletes vitamin C and creates the need for extra antioxidants.

Stress
depletes several of the vitamins and minerals, particularly vitamin B group and C, and magnesium and zinc. One reason, perhaps, why when under stress we are more susceptible to minor ailments.
That downward spiral again!

And It's Not Just *What* You Eat . . .
How and when you eat can affect your energy levels almost as much as what you eat, so here's a guide to planning your meals to maximize vitality and minimize sluggishness.

• Avoid large meals, particularly ones high in carbohydrates. Your body has trouble digesting a large meal; to cope, blood is diverted from the brain, leaving you feeling fatigued or even sleepy, with mental abilities temporarily impaired. Carbohydrates, particularly bread and pasta, are mild sedatives and so eaten in large quantities will add to the problem.

• Eat little and often. If you want to feel alert all day long, eat several smaller meals evenly spaced throughout the day. Two medium meals, (lunch and dinner), one small meal (breakfast) and two snacks (mid morning and mid afternoon) are ideal. All meals and snacks should contain some carbohydrate, some protein and some fat for optimum blood sugar level control.

• The earlier in the day the meal is, the less 'heavy' carbohydrate it should contain. Fruits and vegetables are carbohydrates, but they are fine because they have a high water content, as are naturally occurring simple carbohydrates, such as lactose in milk and yoghurt, but too high a proportion of bread, pasta or potatoes, rice, cereal or other grains will leave you feeling sluggish for the reasons we've just discussed. A meal with a high proportion of carbohydrates is fine taken in the evening when you have finished work and deserve to relax.

• Don't skip breakfast. You need its nutrients, especially its calories, for energy after the long night's fast. Blood sugar level will be too low for efficiency and energy all morning otherwise.

• Don't go hungry. The one golden rule of eating for energy is, if you feel real hunger, eat a good-quality snack, or build your eating timetable around your most hungry times.

• If you take exercise (which you should be doing throughout the 10-week programme and beyond), you need to bear a few nutrition points in mind to avoid muscle fatigue during exercise and muscle pain afterwards. Eat a high carbohydrate snack an hour before exercising and drink plenty before and during exercise. Again, eat a small carbohydrate snack after exercising and have more to drink. Ideal carb snacks are dried apricots and fresh banana, dried fig and natural yoghurt, rye crispbread with an apple. The 'heavy' carbs - bread, pasta, potatoes, rice, cereal or other grains are fine in moderation either an hour before or soon after exercise.

THE ZEST PLAN

If your diet has recently been particularly poor, with a lot of the energy-robbers, consider this two-day 'Superhealth' Diet to give your body what it needs and nothing else. Follow it for the two days and then move to the main Zest Plan.

Superhealth Diet

This is simplicity itself. All you do is eat and drink as much as you like (within reason – you can even overdose on carrot juice, so don't go crazy on any one item) of the items listed below, over the two days, plus the evening extras and a daily Energy Drink. The only rules are to eat when you are hungry, and to eat 'little and often'. Also ensure that you drink around 2 litres (4 pints) of fluid a day.

Eat or drink what you want of:
- Bottled still mineral water
- Fresh organic fruit and vegetables, raw
- Fresh organic fruit and vegetable juices
- Organic nuts (unsalted), raw
- Seeds
- Organic bio yoghurt or Greek ewes'-milk yoghurt
- Soya yoghurt

Have 1 Energy Drink every morning:
Blend together
250 ml (8 fl oz) skimmed goats' milk or soya milk,
125 g (4½ oz) fresh chopped fruit (e.g. pineapple, raspberries, oranges),
1 small banana,
2 tablespoons yoghurt as above,
1 teaspoon runny honey
1 teaspoon wheatgerm oil.

In the evening on both days have 1 small baked potato in addition to any of the unlimited items above.

The Seven-Day Zest Plan

The Zest Plan is based around those five-star energy foods and all the principles left on 'when and how' to eat. Eating this way should have you feeling satisfied and replete, but also light, energetic, bright and with no 'ups and downs' of energy levels.

Tips
- *Eat organic whenever possible.*
- *Eat food at its freshest and best.*
- *Cook vegetables or fruit minimally, if at all.*
- *Eat freely of the Unlimited Foods listed for the Sizewise Eating Plan on page 26.*
- *Portion sizes aren't stated – eat enough to satisfy your appetite and no more.*
- *Never eat to the point of feeling overfull and/or sluggish.*
- *Eat slowly and chew thoroughly.*

BREAKFAST every day
Either one Energy Drink (see left) or portion of bio yoghurt with chopped dried apricots or peaches, sunflower seeds and a few rolled oats; plus 1 portion fresh fruit or portion bio yoghurt with fruit compote made by simmering a selection of dried fruits, including apricots, prunes and apples, in orange juice until tender, topped with sunflower seeds and oats. Add some chopped fresh fruit before serving.

Two SNACKS every day
Choose two from this list (more if exercising, see guidelines above):
- 2 rice cakes with yeast extract
- 1 portion citrus fruit
- rye crispbreads with a little goats' cheese and 1 fresh fig
- Handful of home-made muesli (containing plenty of nuts, seeds and dried fruit) with a little skimmed milk
- Small banana and bio yoghurt
- Handful of almonds or brazil nuts and 1 peach or nectarine
- Handful of dried apricots or peaches with a spoonful of sunflower seeds

FRESH FRUIT
When fruit is mentioned but not specified within the diet choose any fresh raw fruit but aim to eat plenty of: apricots, peaches, nectarines, melons, citrus fruits, berry fruits and pineapples.

LUNCHES AND EVENING MEALS

DAY 1
Lunch Salad of blanched almonds, dried apricots, mixed leaf salad including minimum of one dark leaf, such as spinach or watercress, plus a ripe avocado, all tossed in olive oil and lemon dressing; served with small amount of rye bread.
Evening Casserole of diced venison or Quorn or tofu chunks with mushrooms, red peppers, fresh vegetable stock and thickened with tomato paste. Serve with chopped green vegetables stir-fried very lightly in sunflower oil; baked sweet potato; fresh fruit.

DAY 2
Lunch Crab salad: dressed crab served with slices of cantaloupe melon, chopped fresh herbs and salad leaves, rye crispbreads; followed by a selection of dried fruits and yoghurt.
Evening Grilled or baked trout or salmon with fresh peas or mange-tout and broccoli; potatoes; followed by fresh fruit.

DAY 3
Lunch Home-made carrot soup made by simmering and puréeing fresh chopped carrots with vegetable stock and tomatoes, seasoned with fresh coriander, sesame seeds and swirled with bio yoghurt; serve with small amount of rye bread and follow with fresh fruit.
Evening Tofu and mixed nut stir-fry with beansprouts, green beans, mange-tout, red peppers and broccoli, lightly stirred in sunflower oil; served with brown rice or other whole grain.

DAY 4
Lunch Salad of goats' cheese with tomato, red onion and chopped garlic, mixed salad leaves, tossed in olive oil and lemon dressing; served with wholemeal pitta bread and followed with fresh fruit.
Evening Home-made vegetable chilli using chopped red chillies, selection of fresh vegetables and pulses of choice, ready-cooked (e.g. pinto beans, lentils, chickpeas), simmered in a base of chopped tomatoes, vegetable stock and onion; served on a choice of grains, e.g. buckwheat, barley or millet; side salad.

DAY 5
Lunch Home-made Lentil and Vegetable Soup (see page 32); wholemeal pitta bread; fresh fruit.
Evening Spanish omelette filled with cooked potato, red peppers, peas and parsley; mixed salad.

DAY 6
Lunch Salad of cooled cooked brown rice mixed with pine nuts and sunflower seeds, banana and cantaloupe melon, plus a little chopped chicken; fresh fruit to follow.
Evening Vegetarian pasta bake using wholewheat pasta, cooked brown lentils, chopped nuts, chickpeas and aubergine with a fresh tomato sauce base and topped with a little grated cheese; served with spinach, broccoli and sweet potato.

DAY 7
Lunch Salad of hard-boiled egg, tuna fish, red peppers, parsley, watercress and green salad items of choice, tossed with olive oil and vinegar dressing; fresh fruit to follow.
Evening Classic bouillabaisse fish stew served with rye bread and side salad.

YOUR LONG-TERM DIET

You may repeat the Seven-day Zest Plan for another week or two, but eventually you will want to devise your own diet. Use the following Superhealth lists to ensure you get a real energy-giving balance.

Five-star Foods

These are foods that you should choose as often as you can because nutritionally they offer great value with few 'downsides'. As an example, potatoes and sweet potatoes are similar in their content of calories, vitamin C and fibre and both are healthy, complex carbohydrate foods. But sweet potatoes are richer in more of the important nutrients than ordinary potatoes are – for example, beta-carotene and vitamin E – so sweet potatoes are on the 5-star list while potatoes are on the 3-star list.

Fruits: all fresh fruits, but particularly citrus fruits, avocados, apricots, peaches, nectarines, melons, berry fruits, figs.

Dried fruits:
dried apricots, peaches.

Vegetables:
broccoli, all green leafy vegetables and herbs; all orange, red and dark green salad items and vegetables; asparagus, onions, garlic and sweetcorn.

Nuts and seeds:
almonds, walnuts, sprouting seeds, sunflower seeds, sesame seeds.

Pulses:
all pulses – beans, lentils and chickpeas and split peas.

Grains:
All wholegrains, especially barley, buckwheat, millet, oats, rice, wild rice and rye.

Others:
bio yoghurt, oily fish, tofu, sunflower oil, linseed oil, rapeseed oil, olive oil.

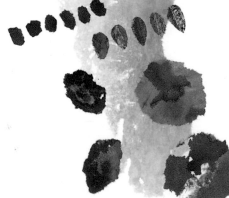

Three-star Foods

These are foods you can add to your 5-star diet to provide variety and extra nutrients and calories.

Dried fruits:
prunes, apples, figs, pears, raisins and currants.

Vegetables:
potatoes, yams (white-fleshed), parsnips, artichokes, fresh beans, aubergines.

Nuts and seeds:
all other nuts and seeds.

Grains and pasta:
preferably wholewheat, noodles, white rice, rye crispbreads, fortified white breads, rice cakes.

Others:
eggs, lean meat and poultry, shellfish, good-quality cheeses (in moderation), skimmed milks, liver and kidneys (unless pregnant), unsalted butter (in moderation), spices, tomato paste.

Other Foods

These are the foods that you don't actually need in order to remain healthy but you may find yourself wanting now and again – the longer you carry on eating the 'Zest Plan' way, though, the less you will have a taste for such foods. If you do keep it to 'now and again' – and 'not much' - you will be fine, but if you allow the quantities of these foods you consume gradually to step up and overtake the high-starred fuel foods above, you will find your energy levels and general health sliding downwards again. *So beware!*

- All highly processed foods;
- All foods containing a list of E numbers;
- All foods high in saturated fat and/or sugar and low in nutrients (e.g. most biscuits, confectionery, pastry, gâteaux, many takeaways);
- Table condiments such as mayonnaise, salt.

SUPPLEMENTS — DO YOU REALLY NEED THEM?

Nutritional supplements are a huge business, from vitamin pills to de-tox drinks. But will any of them really help you to feel better?

If you are eating a healthy nutrient-rich diet like that in the Seven-day Zest Plan here and are in reasonable health, then you shouldn't need a supplement. There are exceptions, however. For instance, if you are in the menopause, or have heavy periods, or continue to smoke, or drink much alcohol, or are under severe stress. But if you think you need a supplement it is best to check with your practitioner first.

Here is a guide to the supplements most often bought to increase energy:

Guarana – hailed as 'the' vitality supplement, but its main active constituent is caffeine (see page 101) and my advice is to leave it alone.

Ginseng – taken for energy and sexual vitality. Unless you have high blood pressure or your doctor advises otherwise, it is pretty harmless and has produced results for many people for many years, so try it if you like. Even if it is simply the placebo effect, so what?

Vitamin E. Supplements may be useful especially for women in the mid years as even in a nutrient-rich diet it isn't easy to get sufficient for your lifestyle. Buy natural vitamin E (D-tocopherol), not artificial (Dl-tocopherol).

Royal jelly – an expensive supplement with little real evidence to support its claims. However, the same advice applies as that on ginseng.

Evening primrose oil – there is evidence that this and starflower oil work to help alleviate pre-menstrual symptoms, especially breast tenderness and bloating. So if this will help you to feel better, and therefore more energetic, it is worth trying. But you need to take it for at least 3 months to see results.

Physical and mental stamina are facilities we tend gradually to lose as we age. Yet this 'slowing down' isn't inevitable. With the right type of exercise – for both brain and body – you can get back the capabilities you had ten, even 20, years ago.

WORKSHOP 14 IMPROVE YOUR STAMINA

Good sleep, relaxation, a good diet and fun in your life can all help your stamina levels in different ways. But the single most important factor is to 'exercise for energy'. You need to improve your cardiovascular fitness, the fitness of your heart and lungs. This heart-lung fitness – or lack of it – has much more far-reaching effects than you may realize.

Here are just some of the ways that cardiovascular fitness – and the activity it takes to get that way – can help you sail through your daily life without feeling drained or exhausted.

• A fit body is better able to cope with all the demands made on it, therefore it gets less tired and you can do more, work harder, and work for longer.

• Your circulation - which is directly linked to the fitness of your heart and lungs – Improves, increasing your metabolic rate, meaning that everything is working faster and you feel more alive and more energetic. It also means, by the way, that you can turn the central heating down because you will naturally keep warmer – and a too-warm room temperature is a major cause of lack of alertness.

• Oxygen uptake improves as your heart fitness and lung capacity improve. As more oxygen and glucose reach the brain, your mental abilities increase, including concentration, memory and reaction time. Research shows that physical exercise helps stop mental decline more effectively than any other measure.

• With heart-lung fitness, increased activity and oxygen uptake, you sleep more soundly and wake more refreshed, so adding to the cumulative effect.

• Increased oxygen uptake and physical activity improve your mood; you feel more cheerful and positive because of natural endorphins released during exercise. Research shows that a positive mood helps stamina by producing extra momentum to help you through boring, difficult or long tasks.

• Aerobic and other forms of exercise help minimize symptoms of PMS and menopause.

Building more exercise into your life

Apart from your 'formal' sessions of aerobic exercise you should begin to build more activity into your everyday life – every little really does help.
• Walk rather than using transport.
• Go as fast as you can up stairs and don't use a lift when stairs are available.
• On holiday, instead of lying on a sunbed make sure to get in at least two active sessions a day – swimming, tennis, dancing – anything that gets your heart and lungs working helps.

Making Your Body Work for You

So how do you achieve cardiovascular fitness, especially if you've not raised a sweat for years? Any one of any age – as long as your health has been given the OK by a physician – can improve cardiovascular fitness to such an extent that you can turn back time. A sedentary person, within 10 weeks of beginning a stamina-building programme, can increase fitness by up to 80%.

All you need to do is regular aerobic exercise suited to your own level of fitness. Aerobic exercise simply means any exercise carried out for a reasonable period of time which raises your pulse (gets your heart beating faster) and causes your lungs to work harder by taking in more oxygen.

And it really is never too late to start. The alternative – to carry on 'slowing down' and do no aerobic exercise at all – will be to condemn your body to old age before you need.

Before you begin an aerobic exercise programme you need to check that you have no contraindications. If you answer 'yes' to any of the following questions, you MUST check with your practitioner before beginning the programme that follows – or any other exercise programme.
• Are you aged 50 or over and have done no formal exercise within the last five years?
• Do you have a Body Mass Index of 30 or over (see Workshop 1)?
• Are you suffering from any medical condition now, or have you recently?

• Are you pregnant or have you given birth within the past six weeks?
• Have you any physical condition that might make exercise difficult (e.g. back pain, arthritis)?

If yes to any, see your doctor and show him this plan. Get his okay. Any of the above contraindications won't necessarily stop you from exercising, but your doctor will probably reassure you by checking blood pressure, heart rate, and so on.

Right – so you have the all clear to exercise. Now we can proceed to the next test, which involves finding out how fit – or unfit! – you really are. For this, all you need to do is walk a measured mile.

The Measured Mile

• Measure out a mile (1.6 km) walk on flat, even ground, using a pedometer or a car (or measure it on a map as a last resort).
• Put on comfortable, cushioned walking shoes, wear comfortable clothes, and warm up by marching on the spot slowly for two minutes. *Make sure you have a watch.*
• Start walking your mile route at as brisk a pace as you can manage without having to stop to get your breath back and while still being able to talk. *If you are walking alone, count to 10 now and then out loud, which will do instead of talking.*

You should feel your heart beating more strongly and should be aware of your lungs working harder to take in more air than normal, but you shouldn't feel real discomfort, such as pain in your chest or lungs, or any burning in your leg muscles. *If you do – stop, and start again, if you feel able, at a slower pace.*
If you can't complete the mile without discomfort – fine, just stop and record how long you did walk.
• At the end of your mile, take note of how long it took you to cover it.

Aerobics for your looks too!

As a bonus, you will find that aerobic exercise will help you look more youthful, too. The extra blood-flow to the skin (through better circulation) will improve your skin's condition, tightening pores, lessening pallor and giving the skin a healthy glow.
Even better, because aerobic exercise burns up calories, it helps you to get, or stay, slim.

Your Fitness Result

	35 *or under*	36 – 55	56+	
Couldn't walk the mile	A	B	C	A = *Extremely unfit*
Took over 20 minutes	B	C	D	B = *Very unfit*
Took 18 – 20 minutes	C	D	E	C = *Quite unfit*
Took 15 – 17 minutes	D	E	F	D = *Slightly fit*
Took 14 minutes or less	E	F	G	E = *Fit*
Took 13 minutes or less	F	G	G+	F = *Very fit*
Took 12 minutes or less	G	G+	G++	G = *Superfit*

Your Fitness Programme

Your main activity during the ten-week programme will be simply to build up your stamina through walking. This is because it is simple, cost-effective, can be done from your own home, requires little special equipment and your progress is easy to monitor.

All I want you to do is go out and walk three times a week (four, if you like, in later weeks) and work through the fitness levels above. For instance, if you are aged 45 and you scored D on the fitness assessment, your goal is to reach G over the weeks ahead. If you are aged 56 and you scored C on the fitness assessment, your goal is to reach F or better. Anyone – yes, anyone – can improve at least three levels during the 10-week programme. Most of you will be able to improve right up to G.

To do this, all you need to do is follow the same instructions given for the Measured Mile test; get out there and walk and gradually your times will improve and as your times improve, you will be getting fitter.

Here are some additional notes before you begin:
- If you already rate an F or G, you are already fit and need only maintain your current level of fitness for adequate stamina. This will entail walking at level F or G three times a week for 20 minutes or more (obviously you will be walking more than a mile in this case). If you do want to increase fitness you will need to provide your body with harder work, which will mean something such as hill-walking, jogging (only advisable in top-quality shoes, on a non-road surface and if you have no joint problems), circuit training in the gym, or cycling, for example.
- Every time you walk, don't forget that to increase fitness you MUST raise your heart rate and feel your lungs working. Work as hard as you can within the 'talk test' level. As long as you keep doing that, you will keep improving.
- Walk with a good style – fairly upright with tummy and bottom tucked in, legs striding out from hips, shoulders relaxed and down, eyes looking forward, not down, arms swinging naturally by sides.
- Don't forget a 2-minute warm-up, and it is a good idea to have a 2-minute cool-down too (the leg stretches on page 37 are also a good thing).
- Once you've worked up to level F or G, you should continue walking after the measured mile to complete a minimum of 20 minutes all together. If you walk for longer than that, you will get fitter more quickly and you will burn extra calories, so don't think of the 20 minutes as a maximum – it's a minimum.
- Most people will be able to progress up one level per 3-6 sessions (1-2 weeks).
Make this your goal.

What to Do When You Can't Walk

What do you do if the weather is too bad to walk, or it's too dark out there? Consider other aerobic options – if your walk really IS off today, it is better to do something rather than nothing.

Here are some first-choice options:
- Invest in an indoor aerobic machine. My favourite is a Healthrider which is no-impact (good on your joints), exercises all your major muscles at once, is quiet and – most importantly – is fun to use. During the winter months I can't remember how I used to get by without it. Other choices are an exercise cycle, a rower or a treadmill.
- Buy a Step. Good lower body and cardiovascular workout like walking and cycling; burns about the same number of calories. You'll need a video to go with it; otherwise it gets boring.
- Buy an aerobics video. There are plenty of good ones for sale – all you need is a reasonable space in front of the TV. Some have routines that are quite hard to follow at first, something to beware of if you have two left feet.
- Buy a mini trampoline (rebounder). Good low-impact exercise, ideal for those with joint problems.

Second-choice options:
- Buy a skipping rope. Fabulous aerobic exercise but if you are unfit very hard to keep up for longer than a minute or two. Also, you need to do it outdoors or in a high-ceilinged room. However if you do persist, your minute session will soon progress to 5 minutes, and five minutes of skipping is very good cardiovascular exercise.
- Stairs. If you have stairs, climb up them at a pace to get your heart rate raised and your lungs working. Keep it up for several minutes.
- Marching/jogging on the spot. If all else fails, march vigorously on the spot for several minutes. Start off at a warm-up pace, then gradually get faster, raising knees higher and pumping arms harder. When you finish, slow down to cool down.

MIND GAMES

Your brain-power will improve as your physical stamina improves but you can do still more to give your mind back its sharp edge. *Try these ideas:*

Give yourself air: your brain needs fresh air so never waste an opportunity to give it some.
Mental exercises. Improve your brain's stamina through the mental equivalent of aerobic exercises. For concentration – turn your book or paper upside down and continue reading for as long as you can. Time yourself. Do it for longer tomorrow. For memory – read a small paragraph in your book or paper once, put it away and try to memorize it. Tomorrow, try to do better. Once you can do one paragraph, make it two. For sharpness – time yourself while you go through the alphabet out loud attaching a word to each letter. Tomorrow, do it quicker. Then do two words to each letter, then three.
Stretch your mind at every opportunity; e.g., instead of buying that sex blockbuster for a journey, think twice – get the novel that will make you think.
Do something different. If you are set in many habits, alter as many as you can; e.g. you always follow the same pattern when you get up. Alter it. You always read the paper in a certain order. Alter it. You always go to the same supermarket and shop in the same order. Go somewhere else. If your mind is fed the same diet it loses its powers of enquiry and observation.
Supplement? Gingkho Biloba and L-Carnitine are two supplements said to improve mind stamina and energy. Taken as instructed they should have no side effects so you may like to give them a try.

H ow long is it since you last really relaxed? One of the greatest energy-sappers of all is a state of near-permanent stress and yet for very many women, that is how they live their lives. This workshop is concerned with teaching you to wind down and let your body, and your mind, recharge their energy levels.

WORKSHOP # 15 LEARN TO RELAX

T he longer you spend without relaxing, the harder it becomes. Also, the more it shows in your looks. A recent major British study concluded that women subject to a period of anxiety began to look older within months, but if they could be taught to relax and avoid stress, they began to look younger again.

First Relax Your Body
These are all symptoms that you need to relax your body:

• Frown lines

• Tight scalp

• Area where skull meets neck sore when gently pressed

• Shoulders up high, knotted muscle easily felt either side of neck

• Teeth clenched, jaw stiff

• Voice high, hoarse

• Fingernails digging into palms .

• Physical nervous habits – e.g. hair twisting, nose scratching

• Shallow breathing

• Fast pulse-rate without exertion

• Difficulty in taking a deep breath

• Toes bunched up inside shoes

• Heartburn

• Nails bitten

How many of those symptoms is your body displaying now? The more you have to own up to, the less relaxed you are. These physical symptoms are just that – symptoms of your unrelaxed mind and unrelaxed lifestyle. Nevertheless, rather like unravelling a ball of yarn, you need to teach your body to relax first – then tackle the problems causing that tension.

Through Exercise

As we saw in Workshop 14, physical activity is a great giver of energy, turning a lethargic body and a slow mind into energized vital ones. But almost as importantly, it is a wonderful natural relaxant. If only everyone who uses tranquillisers, sleeping pills, alcohol or drugs in their attempts to relax would just try regular exercise first!

Exercise works to relax you in several ways. Aerobic exercise releases natural endorphins that improve your mood. It also warms your body up – a similar effect to taking a 'relaxing' hot bath. And it disperses a build-up of adrenaline common in people who are stressed out. The adrenaline builds up in response to stress as your body prepares to 'fight or run', but in modern life our fights are more likely to be verbal than physical, and we don't run away – so the adrenaline stays in our bodies. As aerobic exercise mimics 'fight or run', it works perfectly to calm us down.

A period of exercise in a different environment – say, walking – also gets you away from whatever it is that is tensing you up and gives you time to cool off and calm down. Lastly, if you are tense, you hold your muscles taught and tense and lactic acid builds up in them, causing aching and stiffness and making it hard to relax the muscle without help. Activity of the right kind – say, a stretching session – can release those muscles.

The 10-week programme includes, for everyone, regular aerobic activity and a stretching session to finish your Total Tone routine three times a week. The long body stretch (see page 51) is a wonderful tension releaser at any time but if you scored very high on the list of tension symptoms above, you may want to build more relaxing exercise into your daily life. Here are some guidelines:

• Take your aerobic exercise at a time of day when you are most likely to be stressed – e.g. if you wake in the morning feeling tense about the day ahead, take your walk then. If a bad day leaves you tense, the activity taken then will help you to relax through the evening. The 10-week programme suggests aerobic exercise three times a week, but you can increase this (once you are fit enough to cope) to up to 6 times a week.

• On days you are not doing the Total Tone routine, do the Warm-up and Cool-down stretches one after the other, twice a day. This will take you about 8 minutes a session. Once you are used to the stretches you can do them for longer.

• Consider adding a regular yoga session into your schedule. Yoga relaxes mind and body at the same time and creates energy.

SIX INSTANT WAYS TO RELAX

❶ **Clench your jaw** by biting teeth hard together. Now open your mouth as wide as you can and say 'aaaah'!

❷ **Sigh** as loudly and deeply as you can then take in a good breath of fresh air.

❸ **Smile.** Even better, laugh. Laughter is a physical and mental relaxer.

❹ **Do a few neck rolls** – sit with spine upright and shoulders as relaxed as you can get them. Now slowly roll your neck down towards your right shoulder as far as it can go, return to the top and roll down to the left. Repeat 5 times.

❺ **Shrug your shoulders** – with arms at your sides, lift your shoulders up towards your ears as far as they will go, then pull them down as far as they will go. Repeat 5 times.

❻ **Face massage** – starting above the inner eyebrows and using first and second fingers of both hands, gently make small circular motions (clockwise with your right fingers, anti-clockwise with your left), gradually moving your fingers across your forehead to the temples then, even more gently, down beside your eyes and in across the cheekbones to your nose. Feel those tension lines around your eyes disappear!

Through Massage

For thousands of years the relaxing benefits of a good body massage have been appreciated. Massage works by, first, literally calming the nerve receptors in the skin, then by decreasing blood pressure and pulse rate, by promoting removal of lactic acid in the muscles and by inducing deeper breathing and a sense of well-being. I believe that even if a woman can afford neither the time nor the money for any other luxury or perk in her life, she should make the time and find the money, if necessary, for a regular massage session.

If you feel too guilty for such indulgence, perhaps Section Three – and particularly Workshop 24 – will help you to change your mind. However, even if you don't pick up the phone and book that massage course, you can sample its benefits with a short self-massage explained below. Even better, if you have a partner you can try techniques out on each other.

It is also well worth learning the basics of reflexology - a form of massage it is relatively easy to carry out on yourself.

Self-massage

Work on your 'trigger points' – those painful nodules caused by stress leading to a muscle spasm, reduction of blood flow to the area and build up of lactic acid. Using finger pressure, you can disperse the lactic acid, get the blood flowing again and thus relax the muscle. Use finger pressure as firm as you can bear and hold each press for a slow count of ten unless otherwise stated. Don't use massage oil.

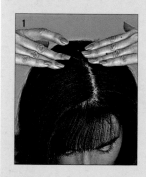
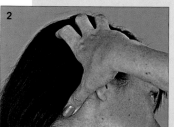
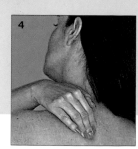

1. Use the third and fourth finger of each hand to press the crown of head.

2. Using your thumb, press at one-inch intervals along the base of the skull, first one side and then the other.

3. Using left-hand fingers, squeeze right side of neck, then use right-hand fingers on left side of neck.

4. Use right-hand fingers to press the muscle at the back of the left shoulder in the triangle between collarbone and shoulder-blade, as shown. You will immediately know when you have found the right spot! Repeat on the other side.

5. Move fingers slightly further in towards spine and press again. Repeat to other side.

Reflexology

In reflexology, pressure is exerted with the fingers or thumbs on reflex points in the feet that are said to correspond to different parts of the body. The toes correspond to the head and neck and then the farther down towards the heel of the foot that you progress (along the sole) the nearer you get to the lower body.

If your neck is tight, the inner side and base of your big toe will be very sore when pressed; if your shoulders are tense the ball of your foot just below the little toe will be correspondingly sore. To work the spine, press all along the inside edge of each foot, from big toe to heel, following the line of the arch of the foot. But an all-over foot massage, five minutes each foot using firm pulsing finger or thumb pressure at 1 cm (½ inch) intervals, is very relaxing in itself – we don't give our feet enough attention and to have them 'worked over' is a real pleasure.

To do self-reflexology, sit on the floor or bed with legs crossed. Use the right hand to work the left foot and vice-versa, and use the non-working hand to hold the foot firmly. Hold the heel if working the toe area and the toes if working the heel or mid foot. If you find a particularly tender area, give it extra time.

Through breathing

If you are tense you are likely to be breathing very shallowly and too quickly, which means that your body will not be getting enough oxygen – a symptom of which is, ironically, anxiety. Your lungs will not be expelling the waste – gasses, carbon dioxide – efficiently, either, a symptom of which is fatigue. This self-perpetuating vicious circle needs to be broken if you are to feel better. Deep correct breathing can calm you down within minutes and will also energize you.

If possible, lie down with loose clothing, on your own. Exhale as long as you can, through the mouth. Inhale to a count of ten through the mouth, feeling your diaphragm (under your ribcage) and your abdomen rise. Really try to get in enough air to fill your lungs completely. Now slowly exhale, to a count of 20, trying to push every last drop of air from those lungs. Try this for two or three minutes.

When you go about your normal life, keep remembering – give yourself oxygen! Get rid of all that carbon dioxide!

BREATHE!

These are all symptoms that you need to relax your mind:

- You skip from one chore to another without completing any.
- You can't concentrate on reading.
- You can't 'switch off' your mind at the end of the day.
- You worry about small things that don't bother other people.
- It doesn't take much to make you lose your temper.
- People tell you things but they don't seem to arrive in your brain.

There's a lot going on inside your head – but that's not necessarily a good thing! If you said 'yes' to more than one of the above list, it's time to calm down, clear your mind of all the rubbish and relax. Long-term, you need to look at your lifestyle and reorganize it so you don't keep going into 'overload' (Workshops 12 and 17–24 will help), but short-term there is also plenty you can do.

At least once a day, you need to make time for yourself, time in which you will use your own responses and outside methods to help you relearn the technique of mental relaxation.

Reduce outside negative stimuli

Here are some of the outside stimuli that may be adding to your mental tension:

- Loud, noisy music of a type you don't enjoy.
- People shouting or talking too loudly, especially about something you find distasteful or boring.
- Television on too loud.
- Traffic noise.
- Bright lights, particularly flashing.
- Insistent noise – e.g. hammer hitting, road drill.
- More than one person trying to talk to you at the same time.
- Crowded space, e.g. in a train, at a party.
- Phone ringing constantly.

Many of us live with negative stimuli like these every day of our

Now Relax Your Mind

lives and don't realize what a huge impact they have on us. Some you can perhaps alter; others aren't so easy to do anything about. But what you need to do is find that time at least once a day to create your own positive, calming environment.

Increase outside positive calming influences

Create your own calming environment by using one or several of the following suggestions:

- blackout eye-mask and earplugs to counteract negative noise/sight stimuli.
- Use personal audio instead of earplugs to listen to relaxing music or sounds you do enjoy. The 'New Age' tapes and CDs of people such as Philip Chapman, Medwyn Goodall and John Richardson are ideal.
- Walk in a pretty and quiet place. Even in the middle of a city there are parks and gardens for you to enjoy.
- Make your own retreat. Create one place that is for you and you alone to relax in and enjoy. A corner of a room if not a whole room, a hut in the garden or, if you have nowhere, make the bathroom your refuge. Inside your refuge always push worrying thoughts away and practise letting your mind float. Allow only good thoughts to intrude. Breathe deeply.

TRY A RETREAT

Why not try a week at a retreat this year for your vacation, or if you haven't that much time, a weekend? Retreats are geared to stress reduction, relaxation, peace and healing. You will find exercise, massage, counselling and more at most retreats and the cost is usually much less than that of health farms or beach hotels.
In the UK, get The Good Retreat Guide (Rider £11.99) or phone leading retreat specialists Stop the World (0171 228 0463).

- Try Flower remedies such as Bach White Chestnut or Rock Rose to help you relax, or use herbalism – hypericum is a good mind relaxer. Or the essential aromatherapy oils ylang ylang, valerian, camomile and lavender applied in firm stroking movements to your forehead and chest will calm you down. The homeopathic remedy arg nit. is worth trying, too.
- Use colour. Avoid rooms or clothes in red, purple, orange. Blues and greens are the most soothing colours – another reason why a walk in the country is relaxing.
- Use food – a diet high in potassium and carbohydrates is a calming one. Try extra bananas, bread, watercress and celery.

Learn to focus

The unrelaxed mind is likely to be focusing on too many things at once. Learn some techniques to help you focus on one thing at a time.

- Decide on paper, in what order you are going to tackle things and train yourself to stick to the order. At first you may only be able to do the first two things on the list in a focused, orderly way without straying. Gradually, however, if you keep focusing every day you will improve.
- Use meditation. During your quiet time of day (see above), sit and relax as much as possible and breathe deeply. Focus your eyes on a point ahead of you. Clear your mind of everything. If a thought comes into your head, banish it (try putting it in an imaginary balloon and letting it float off above your head and out of the room). Think of a relaxing word for you and keep repeating the word. Meditate for five minutes or longer.
- Count down from a hundred. See how far you can get before an extraneous thought comes into your head. When it does, try the balloon trick (above) and start counting from one hundred again. Eventually you should be able to get to zero without losing focus.

Long-term

Long-term, you need to work on the major causes of your day-to-day tension. Your body and your mind are, after all, just reflecting what is going on in your life when they get over-stressed and seize up, or go into overdrive.

Section Three, beginning on page 118, will help you decide what it is you really want and will give you some ideas on how to make changes. Some things, of course, you cannot change; at least not for the moment. Then you should spend your daily 'quiet time' planning for the future in a positive way. But don't be too hard on yourself; and don't expect miracles. You will never be able really to relax if you always feel as though you are one step short of where you really want to be. Perhaps where you are NOW is not such a bad place after all? Use your quiet time to ponder on THAT thought tomorrow.

A good night's sleep ... a simple, natural process; the end result of a busy and tiring day – or something you haven't experienced in ages and would kill for? This workshop explains how to improve your sleep quality without resorting to drugs.

Sleep problems tend to fall into two categories – trouble getting off to sleep when you go to bed, or waking after two or three hours then finding it impossible to get back to sleep. We look at both scenarios here. Check down the ideas and pick the ones that most suit your situation.

WORKSHOP **16** DEEP SLEEP

DON'T . . .

Go to bed if you're not really tired. Stay out of the bedroom until you do feel tired.

Sleep in the mornings to make up for a bad night's sleep. This will disrupt your body clock and make it even harder to get a good night's sleep the next night. It is better to go for one day a little tired, get some outdoor exercise and try all the ideas above to make sure you do sleep well the next night. The odd bad night won't harm you.

Sleep longer than necessary. In the winter it may be a nice idea to cuddle up, turn over and go back to sleep – but if you woke up naturally, it meant you had had enough sleep. Too much will leave you lethargic and likely to have a worse night's sleep next night.

Take sleeping pills except as an absolute last resort. Natural sleep is what you need. And taken more than occasionally, sleeping pills gradually lose their effect in any case, leaving you with few options left, except to take stronger and stronger doses – in other words, they are addictive.

Regular, restful sleep is vital for a healthy and energized body and mind. Lack of sleep severely weakens the immune system and can lead to an increase in severity and number of illnesses. Sleep disturbance can affect concentration, memory and creativity; and, of course, the tiredness that comes with not enough sleep brings a host of its own problems, such as irritability and uneven emotional responses and is also linked with a high proportion of accidents.

A good night's sleep is also vital for youthful looks because, during sleep, extra growth hormones are released, renewing and repairing the tissues and cells of the body, including the skin. Even after one poor night's sleep, physical symptoms begin to show – dark circles and/or puffiness around the eyes, pale complexion – no wonder they call it 'beauty sleep'!

Getting off to sleep

During the day, make sure you take at least one session of outdoor activity – the fresh air and the exercise will both help you sleep. Your brain may be tired but your body needs to be tired, too, in order to sleep well. Follow a routine, beginning in the evening when your work has finished, which will gradually wind you down ready for bed:

● Try to put the day's worries and problems behind you by making a 'to do' list for tomorrow. Decide what you will wear tomorrow and get the outfit ready.

● Eat and drink to help you sleep – a small snack containing carbohydrate, calcium and magnesium around one hour before bedtime will help calm your brain down. A cup of warm milk and a small banana sandwich are ideal. Yoghurt with chopped banana is another idea. Such foods help the production of seratonin in your body – a neurotransmitter essential for good sleep. Don't eat hard-to-digest foods late at night, such as cheese, red meat or pulses. If you like wine, one glass of red wine will act as a relaxant and help you to sleep, but don't drink more alcohol than that as it can severely disrupt sleep later in the night. Avoid stimulating caffeine drinks like coffee, tea, and cola.

● If possible, follow a bath-stretch-and-massage routine before bed (for relaxing essential oils see page 56).

● Check out your bedroom for sleep disturbers and sleep enhancers:

Avoid – an over-hot room (it is nice to go to bed in a warm room, but make sure the heating is set to go off within 15 minutes of your intended sleep time) – a stuffy atmosphere is one of the major causes of restlessness.

Avoid - light. If you have to sleep when it is light, try blackout curtains or an eye mask. Don't leave lights on.

Avoid - noise. Your sense of hearing doesn't switch off when you are asleep and any loud or persistent or sudden noise can wake you. Try to eliminate the causes of noise - ask people to close doors gently, turn music down, talk quietly, etc. If you can't eliminate noise, wear earplugs.

Avoid - an uncomfortable bed. Sounds simple, but many people sleep in bad beds! You spend a third of your life in it, so get one you like. Ditto – pillows. A soft but supportive pillow is important – a hard, lumpy one can keep you awake.

Go for – an open window. Fresh air circulating in the room is very important. If you can't open a window have good air-conditioning.

• Take a herbal drink just before sleeping – an infusion of one teaspoon dried, or two fresh, herbs such as camomile in 150 ml (¼ pint) boiling water, left for 10 minutes and then strained is a good sleep inducer.

• During the menopause and in the week before a period, some women find they sleep badly and this is probably due to hormonal disruption at these times. If this is your problem, try the essential oil clary sage in the bath or mixed with almond oil base as a massage oil. Borage oil (starflower oil) is also good used in the same way. All the other solutions in this workshop will also help you.

• Good sex promotes good sleep, so don't turn your back on your partner even if you feel tired.

One or more of the above measures should be enough to send you to sleep and keep you that way – but if you feel you need extra help, you could try one of the herbal sleep remedies on the market. My favourite is passionflower - sold in the UK by Potters under the name Nodoff. But there are many more you can try, each with it own slightly different formula, though the herbs used most often are valerian, camomile, hops and passionflower. It's a matter of trial-and-error to see which works best for you. A supplement called Kava Kava, available at your health food shop, also works for many people.

Waking in the night

Many people find that they can get off to sleep perfectly well at bedtime but then wake a few hours later and lie there for two, three or more hours unable to get back to sleep. This pattern will certainly be helped by the measures outlined earlier but there are a few extra points worth mentioning:

• High alcohol intake is linked with poor sleep quality, particularly from 3-4 hours after going to bed. So if you're drinking more to help you sleep - forget it. The herbal pills are a much, much more sensible alternative.

• If you wake in the middle of the night at a similar time for more than a few nights in a row, it can become a habit that the body adjusts to, and one that is then hard to break. Try going to bed later, or earlier, or sleeping in a different room for a night or two, to break this pattern.

• Waking in the early hours can be a sign of depression, in which case you should see your practitioner, or it could be unresolved anxieties or worry about a future event waking you up. If these last two are the case, you are likely to wake with a panicky feeling, perhaps with your heart racing. Try to use daytime hours to work through your worries and resolve them. Just talking to someone about them can be a great help. Fears always seem worse in the night when everyone else is asleep and it is dark. If this is your problem, then try taking your herbal remedy when you wake, if it is more than four hours before you are due to get up. If it is only two or three hours before your normal wake time, a better course of action is to get up, move to a daytime room and do something pleasant such as reading, listening to music or watching TV. In summer you could even go out for an early walk. If it is work that is worrying

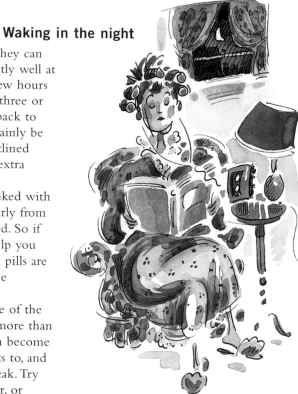

you, you could even try tackling it – the positive feeling you get from having done something constructive about your problem is the first step towards breaking poor sleeping habits for good.

• Shift-work or jet-lag could be causing you to wake at odd hours. In that case you could try taking melatonin tablets to get you back on course. In the UK these are available on prescription only. I wouldn't advise taking them on a permanent basis though, as they have yet to be thoroughly tested long-term for side effects. However they seem to be a better bet than standard sleeping pills.

• Bad dreams may wake you up in the last half of the night, because it is then that you have most rapid-eye-movement sleep, the kind when you dream the most. Some people find they have fewer bad dreams if they avoid caffeine, cheese, chocolate and heavy meals in the evening. If you have many bad dreams that worry you it would be a good idea to see a counsellor.

*P*ositive thought is energy-giving and brings results. Negative thought is enervating and invites failure. It is also ageing and unattractive. So take a lesson in zapping those negative feelings right out of your life.

WORKSHOP **17** # ZAPPING THE NEGATIVES

Are you a negative person or a positive one?

Check out the questions below to find out

1 *You begin a new eating and fitness plan to get in shape but after a week you feel achey and hungry. Do you*

❑ *a.* Give up all idea of getting in shape but feel guilty about it?

❑ *b.* Accept it may have been the wrong plan for you and find a more gentle regime that does suit you?

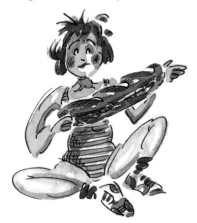

2 *Someone new arrives to live next to you. You take an instant dislike to them. Do you*

❑ *a.* Avoid them and begin house hunting?

❑ *b.* Make a deliberate effort to be friendly and pleasant thinking that they may be giving off 'bad vibes' through nerves or similar?

3 *You're passed over for a job at work because you are not experienced enough. The successful candidate arrives. Do you*

❑ *a.* Seethe inside every time you take an order from him/her and give up trying?

❑ *b.* Be gracious – but twice as determined to get the job you want?

4 *Your ex-husband marries again. Are you more likely to*

❑ *a.* Find yourself bad-mouthing the new wife at every opportunity and refusing to talk to her?

❑ *b.* Try to appear civil and pleased for them?

5 *You are on vacation with two days of your holiday left. Which do you say?*

❑ *a.* Oh, dear, only two days to go; might as well start packing.

❑ *b.* Great – two whole days left, let's see how much we can fit in.

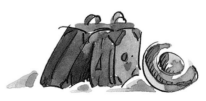

Yes, you know perfectly well! A answers are negative and B answers are positive. Negative thoughts, words, feelings and actions can eat up most of your day if you are not careful – and they can be very habit-forming.

There are two ways to tackle negativity:

1 Act or think positive even if you don't feel it inside. The right feelings often follow.

2 Understand the reasons for your negativity and overcome them.

Let's look at those two points, applied to the types of negativity we experience most often.

Guilt – the women's backpack

Most women are burdened with feelings of guilt at least to some degree. However much you do in your working day, however hard you try to see your friends and look after your family, however many meals you cook or cakes you bake, your efforts never quite seem good enough – so you feel guilty. I even know friends who feel guilty for not giving their cat enough attention or are wracked with guilt because they gave their son ham sandwiches two days in a row for school lunch.

Take this to its logical conclusion and you could literally feel guilty about every single decision that you make in the day. You only put 50p in the volunteer's charity box – guilty! You ate two chocolate biscuits – guilty! You cut short your telephone conversation with your mother, you should have found a better card for your friend's birthday, you only got through half your Open University revision, you weren't pleasant enough to the counter clerk in the bank . . .

Ridiculous really, isn't it? So, first – think positively. Begin to practise turning every negative, guilty feeling and thought into one of pride in yourself. Let's try it with the situations above.

● I am a cat lover. I have a happy, healthy, well-fed cat who gets more attention than most cats I know.

● I make my son a wholesome packed lunch every day rather than letting him buy junk food like some of his friends. Ham is one of his favourite sandwiches.

● I put some money in a charity box today. It wasn't one of my favourite charities, but I like to help people when I can.

● I felt like treating myself so I ate two chocolate biscuits - wasn't I good? I could have had the whole packet!

● I ring my mother most days and talk with her as long as I can even when I am busy.

● I remembered my friend's birthday and sent her a card even though she forgot mine last time!

● My revision was a lot harder than I had anticipated but even so, I managed half of it.

● I had to wait 10 minutes in the counter queue and nearly missed my train but I managed not to take it out on the counter clerk.

So you have turned your negative thoughts into positive ones. And the positive thoughts are MORE valid than the guilt feelings, aren't they? Take an objective view of what you do and you will find that you have little cause to feel guilty. (If you DO have valid cause to feel guilty – for example, if you beat the kids, keep your elderly mother locked up in an attic, starve the cat or habitually rob banks, then you need to alter your behaviour before you can alter your guilt. Ironically, however, truly wicked people rarely feel guilty.

If you aren't the 'guilty about everything' type but have strong guilt feelings about one particular area of

your life – say, you can't see your elderly parents often because you live too far away - consider altering your circumstances to take away the guilt. But look at the pros and cons of such decisions carefully. For instance – if you move to be near them, will you then feel guilty because you are far from your grandchildren? When you have to make a decision based on a 'best compromise', stick with it and use the 'positive thoughts' technique to feel good about the decision you have made.)

Why, then, do you allow so many guilt feelings to ruin your confidence and sap your energy? Guilt without cause is pointless. Look back and see if you can find the answers – they could go back to your childhood; how your parents treated you, how lovers treated you. If you haven't been appreciated enough you will have been trying to be perfect so you can be loved. To delve into such feelings you might like to have counselling. But you don't necessarily NEED counselling to find the cure.

Keep turning those negative guilty thoughts into positive ones and gradually you will feel more confidence and more pride in yourself and your achievements. You will appreciate yourself. And that is a vast lesson to learn.

Handling anger

Anger is not necessarily a negative emotion – it can be useful to kick-start you into doing something that needs doing (e.g. writing to the council to complain about a dangerous road). But if you feel a lot of anger a lot of the time you need to examine the cause(s) and deal with them. Expressed anger is negative for the people on the receiving end; repressed anger is negative for you and bad for your health and energy. Women are usually bad at expressing anger and good at repressing it.

Write a letter to yourself explaining what it is that is making you angry. Many women feel anger because they feel used or abused, taken for granted or helpless in a given situation. Your local women's group can offer advice on who can help you – and Section 3 may give you some answers, too.

Envy – the 'eat you up' emotion

Envy – and its relatives, bitterness and resentment – are the most negative of all emotions. You want what someone else has – a good job, wealth, a particular house, a painting, a talent, a man, a physical attribute, a certain personality, an ability to attract friends. . .

If you find yourself envying somebody anything they are or have, remember the two-point plan.

First, think positively by using what I call 'trade off' technique. Instead of thinking of the thing it is they have that you want, think of something you have that you wouldn't want to change; e.g. 'I really covet her long legs but I wouldn't swap my eyes or my hair.' Focus on the things he or she might envy YOU for. Focus on all the positive sides of your life and if you do it often enough your envy will diminish. You can't be a copy of someone else – and if you could, you wouldn't want to be.

Second, understand that a cause of envy is often that you aren't investing enough time, thought and planning to making your own life work. So stop envying – start planning. Start on strategies for banishing boredom, for improving your looks (well, you're doing that already with this programme), for getting the career, learning the talent, or whatever it is that you envy in others. There may indeed be some things that are beyond your limits for now – but there will be plenty you can do. Use Workshops 18 to 24 to help you.

You can use these same techniques to help banish another emotion similar to envy – a general feeling of dissatisfaction with your life, your surroundings, your 'lot'. You haven't focused your dissatisfaction by using someone else as a role model, but the basic negative emotion is still the same. Think of the positive sides of your life and take action to improve the rest.

Facing your Fears

As we get older, we have more to lose, I suppose. That's why we get to appreciate the familiar things and begin to fear some of the rest. It's no wonder we feel fear. A little fear for the future is a good thing because it makes you appreciate what you have now. But when fear overtakes you and stops you from enjoying the moment or from making changes, it needs taming. This three-point plan will work.
On a piece of paper, divide your fears up into three:
1 Fears that may never happen (e.g. something dreadful happening to one of your children, your partner leaving you).
2 Fears that will definitely or almost definitely happen (you will get old, your pet will die before you).
3 Fears connected with your lack of self-confidence (how will you get through that retraining programme, that speech you have to make).
Now make the positive thoughts for each fear. E.g.
'I am doing everything I can within reason to prevent anything awful happening to my children'
'I am going to get old but I know many fulfilled and healthy older people.'
'I have been accepted on this course/asked to make this speech, therefore I can do it.'
Now try to understand why you have these fears. For instance, if you have a lot of fears in group one – fears that may never come true – you are deeply insecure and you need to tackle the reasons for that. You may need counselling to help you see the future as something good and exciting rather than bleak and worrying.

If you have a lot of fears in group two – usually connected with the natural passage of time – the best cure is to make absolutely sure that you are doing everything in your power to make the most of the people, the places, the times that you value so much now. Make sure you give love and thought and time and appreciation and take what is offered gladly. Grabbing the moment now is an action you can take – and action beats fear.

If you have a lot of fears in group three you need to strengthen your self-confidence. Partly this will come through doing what it is you fear. The more you turn away from things you fear the harder it gets to do them next time, the smaller your world will get, and the smaller your self-esteem.

Last word . . .

There are, of course, other negative emotions – plenty of them – that can sap your energy and upset your life. If you find yourself being negative in any situation, use the three-point method to try to get yourself back to a positive frame of mind. Remember, positivity is an energy source, and energy leads to a fulfilling life. But conversely, a fulfilling life can also GIVE you energy – and the next section, Life Choices –the Inner You, examines all the ways you can make your own life more fulfilling.

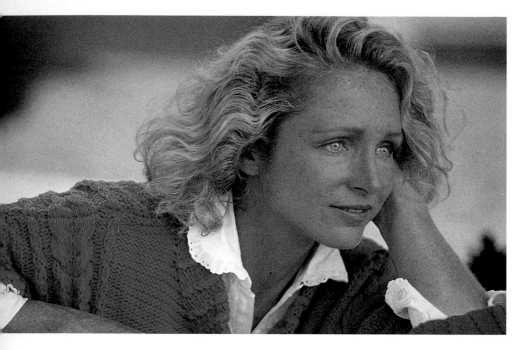

LIFE CHOICES
The Inner You

This section is all about the possibilities in your life. Finding out what they are, which of them you really want, and turning them into reality.

One of the most important differences between youth and old age is that young people dream, plan, plot, 'go for it' – and if something doesn't work out, then they move on to something new without too much regret. At least they tried! Old people don't do this. Or, at least, the older we get the less inclined we are to do so. We tend to put on blinkers and life's possibilities narrow because of that. Attitudes harden, dreams get forgotten. But it doesn't need to be like that.

In our middle years, we can stay young in spirit if we hold on to that youthful mobility of thought, and by never letting a year of life go by without taking stock and planning new things. It's not just new things you need in life; you also need to look at the familiar to see how you can improve your quality of life there too.

In this section you will be doing all you can to revive your enthusiasm, restore your confidence and zest for life, and re-evaluate your position, your values, your needs and your relationships.

Whether you're bored with your job and fancy a complete change, or just feel it's time for promotion – or whether you haven't worked for years and want a new start but feel out of touch, here's how to revamp your career potential for the 21st century.

WORKSHOP **18** NETWORKING

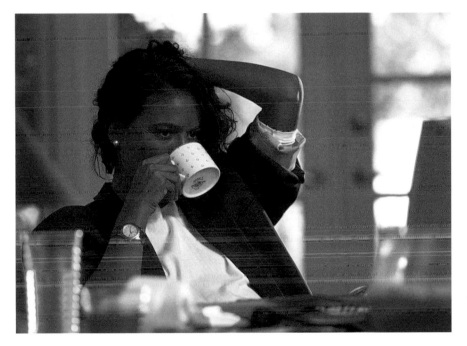

If You've Been Out of the Marketplace for Years

If you haven't worked in a long time, of course the first two things you need to decide are what you would like to do and what action you need to take to secure such a job. You should also have been following the complete 10-week programme, because in the job marketplace your appearance, your health, your confidence levels and everything else that the programme has been designed to help you with, are all-important in helping you secure that new position. If you're competing for a job against 25-year-olds you have many advantages over them – don't spoil your chances by falling down on things like style, over which you have complete control.

If for any reason you haven't been following the programme – start now.

Work that keeps you young. . .

- Work that involves seeing plenty of new faces all the time and talking to lots of people.
- Work that stretches your mind.
- Most work in communications.
- Most work in media.
- Physically active work.
- Work involving travel.
- Work with plenty of paid holiday time.
- Well-paid work.
- Work that requires you to look good all the time, be a role model.
- Work that you enjoy.

Work that makes you feel old . . .

- Working alone all the time.
- Poorly paid work.
- Work that involves very long hours.
- Shift work.
- Repetitive work which doesn't involve the brain.
- Work you live with even at weekends and holidays.
- Work where everyone else is a lot older than you.
- Work in a depressing, gloomy building.

Deciding What You'd Like to Do

You may already have a definite idea about what you want to do. That's fine – with one reservation. If it is what you used to do, maybe 10 or 20 years ago, ask yourself – do I still want to do that? Or am I just going for the safe cosy option and are there other things I could look at? You aren't quite the same person you were then; the job probably isn't the same either. So don't rush too quickly into the same type of work – even to the same company – without thinking it through.

If you don't have a definite idea you need to think big and then gradually narrow the field down to a few ideas that need investigating more thoroughly. Follow this five-point plan:

CASE HISTORY

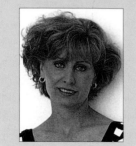

Hilary, 43, left school, got married and had her first baby by the time she was 18.

Three years ago, with Amanda growing up, Hilary realized that she had many years ahead of her and wanted to work.

'I knew I didn't have the skills necessary to work in an office – I wasn't computer-literate, for example. And anyway, the idea of office life didn't appeal to me.'

Instead, Hilary decided that what she really wanted to have was a career in child-care. 'I decided to apply for a course to get my NNEB – to be a nursery nurse. The thought of going to college at my age – then 40 – was quite frightening but I realized that if I didn't train, I wouldn't get the kind of job I wanted. On my first day at college, I passed my lecture room and felt so daunted that I almost didn't go in. But I did - thank goodness – and within a few weeks I felt good about myself. I was proving I still had a brain. Now I have a job I love and the future looks good. When you've spent so long bringing up children it's hard to re-adjust when that job is more or less finished. But you can't sit and do nothing. You've got to make a new life for yourself.'

Gathering ideas

1 Decide into which broad band your ideal work comes. For instance, you may want to work in commerce. You may want to work in the leisure industry. You may want to work in one of the traditional professions – medicine, law, etc. You may like the idea of retail. You may want an outdoor job, or one working with children or animals. You may want to break into media, or work in the social services. You may want to work from home, and/or start your own business (in which case, see Your own Business below). If you're not sure of your 'broad band', the library, bookshops, internet, local careers office, will all help you. Alternatively, you could go on a vocational guidance course – one- or even half-day courses are available. Just because you haven't done something before, that doesn't mean you can't start now – though the more ambitious you are the more likely it is that you will need college training/retraining.

2 Bear in mind your existing talents and interests, and any previous career experience, and see how many of them you could employ in your chosen 'broad band', or which would help your application for a job. If the answer is 'nothing' you may have picked the wrong band. If you're still not sure, carry on to 3.

3 Narrow the broad band down to specifics. For example, if you decided you want to work in the leisure industry, do you want to run a hotel or work in a travel agency or help vet holiday hotels and destinations for one of the big travel companies? If the latter idea appeals to you, it would help if you have much experience of travelling, staying in hotels, writing reports, and so on.

4 Find out whether the type of job you like is available in your area. If not – would you move?

5 Find out (again using the information services above) what qualifications you would need for your ideal job; whether you can get them while working your way through a company (age may be an important factor here) or whether you need to study, or train at a special college or course. Alternatively, write to specific companies or trade associations in your chosen area asking for career/training information.

YOUR OWN BUSINESS

Many women dream of running their own business or of working for themselves from home. Here are some ideas to help make that a reality for you:

● Have a clear idea of what you want to do, how you are going to do it, and ensure you have the aptitude/talent/experience for it.

● Ensure that there is a suitable gap in the market.

● Unless you have unlimited finance and enjoy high-level stress, start small. One idea is to start in a very small way while still in other employment – e.g. if you want to design knits, do it to begin with by word of mouth in your spare time and as you get more orders, think about advertising, giving up work, and so on.

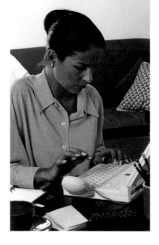

● If you really need backing, go to the bank with a professional proposal covering your plans for the next 2 years with plenty of information on why there is a need for what you are going to offer.

● Work out of your home if at all possible – this immediately cuts costs tremendously.

● If you do work from home, it's important to stay in touch with people – not just customers or clients – to stay sane and happy. *In the UK the organization for the self-employed at home is Breakthrough,(0181 749 8525)*

What Action Do You Need to Take?

Now you need to do what you have to do to get that job.

• If you need to train or pass exams to stand a chance, you need to decide whether you can do that – is it practical for you? Can you afford the time? Can you afford the expense? Investigate this as far as you need to go, even down to visiting the college, say, and talking to the prospective tutor, or whatever.

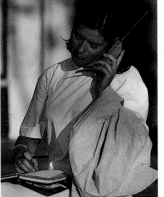

• If cash is a problem, investigate local or national grants, or grants from the company for whom you wish to work.

• Think about starting part-time or job-sharing or doing voluntary work in your chosen profession or job, if appropriate, and especially if you are interested in a job where an immediate full-time paid vacancy is not going to be easy to get. Once you become a familiar face and prove your worth you will find your goal easier to achieve.

• If you know the kind of job you want and that you don't need training, but you don't have a specific company in mind, scan the job advertisements in your papers, local and national, and also in specialist publications, if appropriate (say you want to go into grocery retail, in the UK buy *The Grocer* magazine) and apply for jobs you think may suit.

• If appropriate get a CV organized. You can buy a book on writing a good CV or you can pay to get one professionally done by one of many companies offering this service in the broadsheet small ads. Even if you think you haven't done a great deal over the past years, a good CV writer will certainly make it look as if you have!

• If you get an interview, take a few precautions to help it go well:

Do your homework! Make sure you know all about the company, and rehearse well what you think you could give the company. Make your age a plus, not a minus, by showing maturity, wisdom, experience, self-confidence and poise, as well as good grooming and approachability.

Control nerves by deep-breathing techniques (described on page 110).

Choose a good day if possible, for you to go along to the interview, e.g. after a long weekend break when you are fresh and relaxed; and not at a bad time, such as before a period if you get PMS, or in the middle of a bout of flu.

Wear clothes appropriate for the job – usually smart, slightly understated garments and shoes that make you feel good are the ideal. Avoid anything uncomfortable and avoid anything sexy unless you happen to be applying for a job that requires sexiness.

Have a sense of humour. It's not always easy to strike the right balance, but if you can make them smile it always helps – as long as your humour isn't at their expense or that of the company!

If You're Dissatisfied with your Current Job

Due to the recession, many women I know have stayed in the same job for years, with the philosophy that they are lucky to have a job and daren't push their luck by trying for promotion, moving or trying something totally different. This is a pity. If you use your common sense – and much of the advice above for new job hunters – you can get out of your career rut without risking anything at all.

If you are looking for promotion, or perhaps a sideways move in your current company, you need to be positive, be confident, be determined and also keep your ears and eyes open for opportunities to make your wishes known (if appropriate) or to get considered along with other applicants. You should unashamedly seek out anyone of influence in your company and cultivate them by any fair means – shared lunches, invitations, help with projects, flattery, whatever (don't feel guilty about this, everyone else does it, so you must as well if you are to stand a chance!).

If you are often passed over for promotion in favour of new employees or younger employees, you could either directly ask why and then, if appropriate, work towards improving so that next time you won't be, or you could begin to apply for new jobs. It's best to do this without acrimony as you may well need a reference.

If you decide to apply for a completely different type of job, either within your own 'broad band' or in another, go back to the beginning and use the advice for women who haven't worked in a while.

L *earning isn't just for the young – all research shows that our brains*
stay keener if they are worked and stretched throughout life.
If you haven't really learned anything since you were at school or college,
now is the time to start educating yourself again.

WORKSHOP 19 EDUCATION

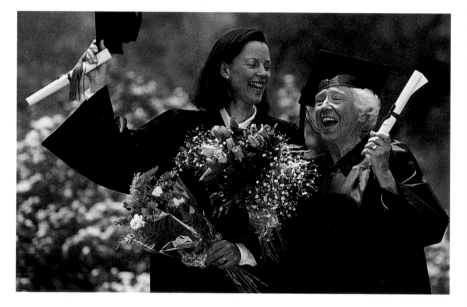

After the frenetic 20s, when you're busy forging a career (and, no doubt, have had enough of books and theses for the time being anyway), and the non-stop 30s when you're coping with children as well as work, your middle years can be the perfect time to rediscover your intelligence and set it to work on new subjects.

It has been said that our learning capacity slows down as we get older – for instance that you can learn the basics of a new language in hours at 12 but weeks at 50. I am sure that is not true. Now you have the obvious advantage of being able to choose to learn something you really want to learn – rather than having something dumped on you at school or college. Wanting to learn, being really interested in your subject is the most important criterion for success. You also have the advantage of experience, and the self-discipline so often lacking when you are a child or young adult.

In this workshop I offer some ideas on what you might like to learn and how you might go about it.

What do you want to know?

• You might like to go back to a subject you liked at school or college and take it further. Spend a few minutes thinking about what you enjoyed or felt you had an aptitude for. A few ideas include: comparative religion, a science, a language, literature, social history, politics, nutrition. Don't take too broad a subject, e.g. in literature try a particular country's work or a particular period in time.

• You might like to investigate one of the subjects you didn't study in full-time education. For instance, when I was at school I remember having to make the choice between history and art. I didn't want to choose between the two but was forced to choose history. In recent years I've tried to make up for that lost subject – not by painting but by studying the lives of some of my favourite artists. Other subjects just weren't around 20 or 30 years ago – what about learning Chinese or doing computer studies, or late twentieth-century literature?

• Most of us have an area in our minds filled with things we'd like to know more about if we ever find the time. Now is the time to go through that mental list and pick something that's been a growing interest for the past few years. Maybe astrology or genealogy; maybe botany or cartography. (For more practical ideas and more general things, read the next workshop about exploring your own potential.)

Whatever you choose, pick a subject, and a method of learning it, that will give you the end-result you want. So it' s time to ask yourself a couple of questions:

• Do I want to learn by myself in my own time and at my own pace?

• Do I want a structured course with a recognized examination and certificate at the end of it?

• Do I just want to do this for

fun/satisfaction and don't want a certificate?

• Can I put by an hour or two/an evening/a day/or more a week to pursue my subject?

A course with a certificate at the end is a goal and a motivation to keep going; however that doesn't suit everyone, and you must decide what you want. Whatever time you have to spare, there are often courses to fit unless you choose something very obscure. Here are a few ideas on how you might begin your chosen subject.

For more on practical skills and hobbies, see Workshop 20.

For more on retraining and job skills, see Workshop 18.

Don't forget, if you're going to study you need to bear a few points in mind from the start:

• You need a quiet place to study.
You need quiet time to yourself with no outside hassles.
• You need to have at least a minimal structure for how you study otherwise progress will be erratic.
• Don't study for too long at a time. Your brain will only absorb material well for an hour or two, especially if you are unused to study or the subject is difficult. After that length of time, take a meal break or a walk or at the least, work on a different aspect of your subject. As you progress you may find you can study for longer – that's your brain stretching as it is worked, which is where we came in!
• Unless you are studying for a certificate in order to get into a new career, you may ask yourself, 'What is the point of me doing this?' The answer is simple – you are doing this for your own satisfaction, to increase your self esteem by proving you can do it, for pleasure, and because life is for learning – don't keep the blinkers on.

Going About It

Especially if you're not sure what you want to study, it's always sensible to start by going to your library for information on local courses, classes and adult education. When you investigate you might find something you like the sound of that you hadn't thought of before.

• The library will also offer information about organizations, clubs and societies that might help you further, especially if your chosen subject isn't covered by local courses.

• If you want to study by yourself in your own way and time without a structure, again the library is a good starting point, or your bookshop will provide information about reading material on its microfiche. CD ROM is useful for visuals. The Internet is also useful if you are disciplined in using it.

• If you opt for regular attendance at a class, promise yourself at the beginning that you will attend every lecture. A good way to do this is to pay in advance for a whole course/year/term, or whatever.

• Private lessons are another option – good for languages and if you are better on a one-to-one basis or can't travel.

• The Open University is ideal for most people and a good compromise between working on a course and doing your own thing.

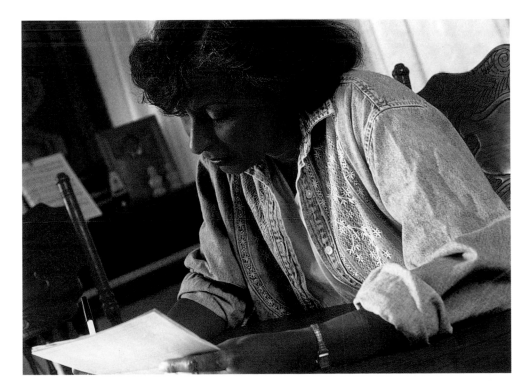

I n this workshop, I want you to be an explorer. No, that
doesn't mean spending your life-savings on travel, or
doing a solo round-the-world tour by elephant. For
certain, travel can be brilliant exploration if you keep
your eyes and your mind open. However, you can – and
many people do – travel and discover nothing. You can
also explore without leaving your own vicinity – and that
is what this workshop is about - exploring your own
potential and life's possibilities. If you lose that ability to
question, search, keep an open mind – then you're old,
whether you're 30 or 100. First try the quiz below.

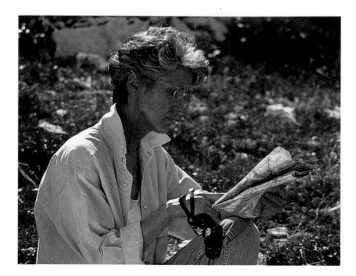

WORKSHOP **20** EXPLORATION

How Open-minded Are You?

Tick the box for each question then check your score on the right.

	often	sometimes	never
1 Could you be persuaded to go to a concert or a play that you think you may hate?	❏	❏	❏
2 Do you enjoy being in the company of people more learned, experienced, travelled or talented than you?	❏	❏	❏
3 On a train, plane, or in a queue, etc., do you find yourself deep in conversation with a stranger?	❏	❏	❏
4 Do you take time to browse in a library or bookshop?	❏	❏	❏
5 Do you find yourself questioning the way things are traditionally done/the way you have always done things?	❏	❏	❏
6 Do you daydream when you should be working?	❏	❏	❏
7 Do you make decisions based on instinct, not logic?	❏	❏	❏

Quiz Results

Now look at your ticks.
Score 4 for every 'often',
2 for every 'sometimes' and
0 for every 'never'.
Add your score:

20-28:
You are open-minded, with a great sense of the possibilities of life. You probably don't need this workshop but I can guarantee you'll read it anyway!
10-19:
You sometimes find yourself wishing you could be more daring. You allow your disciplined side to rule you a little too often and are sometimes afraid to take chances that would have been right. Use this workshop to help you open up a bit.
Under 10:
You tend to have tunnel-vision and you're a bit too 'set in your ways'. You don't like to move from your chosen path, which means you're missing out on so much that could enrich your life. I think you're a little frightened of life, even if you don't admit it. Yes, it is important to be focused and disciplined, but you need balance - use Workshop 15 to help you relax enough to be able to enjoy life and use this workshop to help you see what you might be missing.

TEN IDEAS FOR EXPLORERS

*Read through the ideas that follow thoroughly and apply each one in turn to your life. At the end, make a list
of the best ideas for you – and see how many you can fit into your days in the weeks ahead.*

❶ **Keep an open mind.**
If you ever find yourself saying things like, 'THAT wouldn't be any good!' or 'I NEVER do that', stop and think. Why wouldn't it be any good? Why don't I try that? You may be right – but don't be too quick to turn down ideas, and innovations. Sometimes it is good and invigorating for your mind to try a new action plan, or whatever. Also it is good to rethink your views – on politics, religion, or something simple like what food you enjoy – now and then. By reviewing yourself and your actions and those of other people in relation to you (and doing it throughout your life), you keep yourself fresh and up-to-date. It is so easy just to carry on as you always have – it requires less effort. Once you stop making an effort, however, you start getting old!

❷ **Keep your eyes open.**
People look but often don't see. Start looking around you every day. If you live in the city, have you ever noticed the architecture where you walk every day? If you live in the country, have you ever stopped to examine closely the wild flowers. If you used to do it, how long since you last did? Would you know what kinds of tree grow in your road? Look at people. You need never be bored on public transport if there are other people around. You can play the 'people' game – look at what someone is wearing. Who are they? What do they do? Where are they going?

❸ **Explore your own capabilities.**
In the last workshop we considered how you could get back to education – but how about the other areas of your life? When we are young we tend to push ourselves to see what our limits are; as we get older we give up. However, there is no reason to do so. Tell yourself you can do any-thing you want to do – then decide what that is. If you're fitter with the help of our exercise and stamina workshops, perhaps you can try something new for your body – a new sport, or a new active hobby such as dancing. Isn't it time you tried a new hobby or two? Anything from learning to fly a microlite plane to playing chess. . . write a list now of all the things you'd like to do. Or how about thinking of a money-making interest – maybe you could learn to cut hair, or propa-gate plants, or paint. Don't ever sit at home feeling bored - find out what you can do. And don't put up with a dull job – you can cope with a more interesting challenge, so read Workshop 18 and start looking out for something better.

❹ **Explore other people.**
Other people's brain, minds and knowledge are gifts you should use as often as possible. So if you've stopped listening to people, stopped reading books, stopped asking questions and become insular – think again. You should read as much as you can, listen as much as you can (but not to bores) and take any opportunity to absorb information that helps you improve your life. By using other people's knowledge and experi-ence, you grow and improve.

❺ **Explore yourself.**
The other way you grow and improve is to delve into your own mind. Work out what 'makes you tick' and you can set about work-ing on your faults, maximizing your good points, improving how you deal with others and deciding what you want from your life. It isn't selfish to think about your-self. If you find this hard, there are plenty of self-help books and there are all kinds of self-discovery courses available world-wide – the usual is a week-end course. In the UK try Landmark Forum (0171 580 1997) or Insight (0171 706 2021).

❻ **Stop being a spectator.**
Get into the habit of joining in rather than watching. We watch an average of 3 hours of television a day each. What are your favourite types of programme? You love plays – instead of watching them, how about joining a drama club? You love the sports programmes, particularly golf and tennis? Why not join a golf or tennis club? Do you take the children/grandchil-dren swimming but sit there and watch them? Join in.

❼ **Make things happen.**
Somebody will – why not you? Far too many of us sit around waiting for other people to organize things, to contact us, to make the first move, for our luck to change. You can make things happen and you can make your own luck. Ring people. Get involved in local events (a local paper may not be literature but it is full of news and ideas about your own area). You feel bad about local pollution. Don't moan, set up an action group!

Learn to believe in things you want and be persistent. You may not get it all, but you'll have plenty more than if you sit and wait and do nothing.

❽ **Do something different.**
Get yourself out of a rut by making a conscious effort to change long-standing patterns of behaviour. Your partner always mows the grass. Do it yourself. You always wear black. Wear pink. You always get up at 8 am. Get up at 4am on a June day and enjoy the dawn. You always plan ahead. Today, go to the station and decide when you get there where you will go on the spur of the moment. And so on. Think of some ideas for yourself. You'll get a real buzz from a small change.

❾ **Daydream.**
Every now and then let your mind wander. You might get some good ideas. The best times to daydream are before you go to sleep, when you wake up (if you haven't got to get up straight away) and on a train or plane.

❿ **Be a silent stranger**
How long is it since you took yourself off, on your own, to some where you've never been before – even for an hour? It is a real tonic and a wonderful chance for keep-ing your mind and eyes open, to get in the car or on the bus or train – or even to walk a couple of miles – to somewhere totally new. Find a park and sit and observe. Find a café and while away a lunch time watching peo-ple. If you live in a city it's great to go to an area with a different ethnic mix from your own and pick up the different atmosphere. How long since you saw the sea? Go there and be a stranger. Go on – get a map and decide where to go. If it helps, pretend you're researching a novel or a play. You may get the inspiration really to do it!

W ork and routine often dominate huge chunks of our lives so that in time we often forget how very important – and enjoyable – it is to have a good social life. By that I don't mean parties every night – but a circle of friends we can trust and with whom we can share. Having friends, and being a good friend, isn't selfish or frivolous. Being a sociable integrated person can help you stay young and in touch. Friendship is uplifting, reassuring, revitalizing and stimulating – all things you need to feel good about yourself. Being a good friend also helps you feel good about yourself; it raises your sense of self-worth.

WORKSHOP # 21 SOCIABILITY

Friendship Quiz

So here let's take stock of your social life and see if you can make improvements. First do this Friendship Quiz. Tick the answer that seems to be most near the truth in your case.

1 *How many friends do you have with whom you feel completely at ease and to whom you can tell anything?*
- ❑ *a* None
- ❑ *b* One or two
- ❑ *c* Several

2 *How many friends do you have who aren't connected with your work?*
- ❑ *a* None
- ❑ *b* One or two
- ❑ *c* Several

3 *If you had a private party, how many people can you think of that you'd really like to see there (and who would be likely to accept)?*
- ❑ *a* Not enough for a party.
- ❑ *b* Enough for a small party.
- ❑ *c* Enough for a big party.

4 *If you were extremely depressed what would you be most likely to do?*
- ❑ *a* Sit it out on your own
- ❑ *b* Phone the Samaritans
- ❑ *c* Phone a good friend.

5 *How often do you spend an evening/day in the company of friends?*
- ❑ *a* Less than once a month
- ❑ *b* Every two or three weeks
- ❑ *c* At least once a week

6 *Do friends usually ring you:*
- ❑ *a* Rarely – you always ring them?
- ❑ *b* Always – you don't bother to ring them?
- ❑ *c* As much as you ring them?

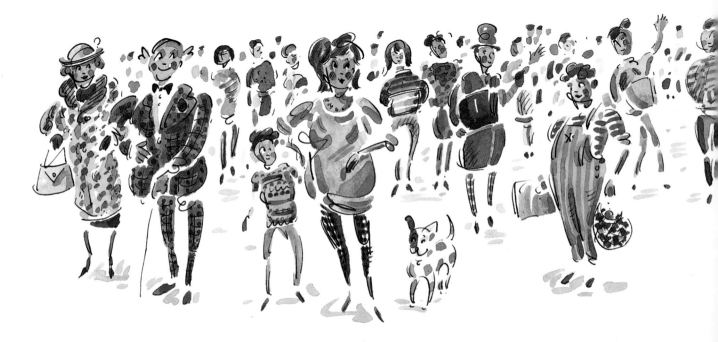

Quiz results

Score 1 for every A, 2 for every B, and 3 for every C you ticked. Add up your score and read your result below.

Over 35:

You're an excellent socializer and no doubt very popular too. You know how to make friends and how to keep them. And you realize how very important they are in your life. You are as good at making deep friendships as you are at making time for people just passing through. You don't really need to do the rest of Workshop 21 (except for page 129) but you probably will - just for fun!

21-35:

You are unsure of your success socially. Sometimes you think you're doing well and feel secure, with enough people you can rely on, and sometimes you're a terrific friend yourself. You can, however, feel a bit lonely and isolated. Maybe you lead a very busy life and find it hard to fit in the demands friends may make on you. It is worthwhile making that effort, though, so do the rest of the workshop and see what areas you most need to work on in terms of your social life.

20 or under:

You want a good social life and close friends and you recognize the importance of both, otherwise you wouldn't have got this far with the workshop. For some reason, however, it isn't working for you. You're likely to lead a quite solitary life (even if on the surface it doesn't appear that way) and have deep bouts of loneliness and maybe even depression. You may also think that self-sufficiency is a quality to be admired, and that reliance on others' attention and affection is a dangerous pastime. The future could be bleak though if you don't loosen up a bit and let more people into your life and your heart. Carry on with the rest of this workshop and really work the ideas through.

---

7 *Are your friends mostly:*

❏ *a* Friends from ages ago; you have no or few new friends?

❏ *b* All new friends, you have no or few friends from years ago?

❏ *c* A mix of old and new friends?

8 *If you move house/change jobs, do you keep in touch with the people you've left behind:*

❏ *a* Rarely?

❏ *b* Occasionally?

❏ *c* A lot?

9 *When you feel like going out, can you find someone to go with you (apart from husband, partner, or family):*

❏ *a* With difficulty?

❏ *b* Sometimes?

❏ *c* Easily?

10 *Do you ever go for days without talking to a friend?*

❏ *a* Frequently.

❏ *b* Occasionally.

❏ *c* Never.

11 *Do you find people boring?*

❏ *a* Yes, many people.

❏ *b* A few people.

❏ *c* Very few people.

12 *Do you remember your friends' birthdays:*

❏ *a* Rarely?

❏ *b* Sometimes?

❏ *c* Always?

13 *Do you have any friends you'd be happy to see you crying?*

❏ *a* No.

❏ *b* Maybe one.

❏ *c* More than one.

14 *At Christmas, how many cards do you get, excluding relatives and business cards?*

❏ *a* Hardly any.

❏ *b* Quite a few.

❏ *c* Dozens.

---

10 WAYS TO FIND NEW FRIENDS

❶ Don't be too reserved. If you like the look or sound of someone, talk to them, find out what they like and when the time is right make a casual invitation based on what you know. For example, she likes gardening – suggest she might like to come along with you to a garden open to the public. Don't always expect other people to initiate a friendship – why should they, after all, any more than you ALWAYS should?

❷ What interests do you have that you could share by joining a club? Singing, acting, gardening, painting, whatever you enjoy there is a club to join. Haven't got any Interests? Of course you have (and Workshops 20 and 24 will help you).

❸ Alternatively, try starting a club of your own – a hobby club, a dining club, a theatre club, whatever.

❹ Join a quiz league.

❺ Ask for help. People like being helpful and it makes them like you.

❻ Offer help. You're good at something other people want to learn; offer your help. Let people know you're glad to help.

❼ Go to college.

❽ If your work is isolating, work a few hours a week somewhere more sociable – say, a shop selling something you enjoy, or a restaurant, or sports club. Many places need extra help at busy times.

❾ Get a pen-friend or two.

❿ Slow down – if you're always in a hurry without time to stop and chat you could lose many opportunities for making friends.

HOW TO KEEP FRIENDS HAPPY

- Ring them regularly.
- Don't feel snubbed if sometimes they are busy with other things.
- Don't always moan – be cheerful at least some of the time.
- Don't tell anything other than occasional white lies, and if you do, ask yourself how you could avoid the white lie.
- Don't be afraid to show your vulnerable side, your failings and failures.
- Listen to what they have to say.
- Only offer advice if you're asked – and then be very careful, especially about saying anything negative about your friend's partner, family, other friends, and so on.
- Remember birthdays.
- Pay your way and never borrow anything without returning it or replacing it.
- Remember, in most situations you can say something negative or positive – the positive is nearly always the right thing to say.
- Don't burden your friend(s) too heavily. You cannot reasonably expect her/him to be there for you every minute of every day at a second's notice.
- Don't expect your friend(s) to want to share all your interests. That's why a circle of friends is a good idea.
- Remember to give as well as take.

Shyness or reserve – or the simple lack of ability to make initial 'small talk' – can be a barrier to making friends, but this needn't be so. Most good friendships are built up through a common interest – whether it is work, having children at the same school, living in the same apartments or sharing a hobby.

Sometimes our lack of a social circle is simply because the life we lead doesn't offer opportunities to meet people. For example, someone who has recently moved from town to country and works from home will have to make an effort to go places and do things to make friendships happen.

The box on the previous page gives you 10 good ways to meet or encourage people who may become friends – look through it and use it. Not all ideas will be possible for you, but some WILL work.

Setting about making new friends in the mid-years is a wonderful challenge. The possibilities are exciting and almost endless, and it's truly never too late to start.

Keeping Friendship Alive

By the time we reach our 30s and beyond, most of us have had many friends in our lives. Most of us, too, have LOST as many friends. Obviously, it's almost impossible to

Making Friends

stay friends with every person you've known throughout your life - but to keep a proportion of your friends throughout life is enriching and even more important than having the knack of getting friendship off the ground.

Do you like people?

I know someone who gets through 'friends' at an alarmingly quick rate – the fallout is tremendous. She will drop someone for any small reason – for example, being late to meet her; not agreeing with her; forgetting to pass on a piece of gossip, or saying something critical.

To be a good friend you need to give as much as you take, and you have to like your friends and be interested in their lives. Even more importantly, you need to accept them with their failings.

No friend is perfect, so don't discard people before you've honestly asked yourself, 'Am I expecting too much?' If you wait for the perfect friend, you'll die waiting.

Do people like you?

What is it that makes one person say of another person, 'I don't like HER!' or, 'I could never be friends with HER!'?

Generally, saying we don't like someone translates to, 'That person makes me feel negative about myself in some way.' We don't like people who make us feel inferior, stupid, dull, invisible, jealous, and so on.

So if you think you are more likely to be popular if you always have the latest car, live in the best house, wear nothing but designer clothes, never have a hair out of place and always want the

last word – you couldn't be more wrong. You are only likely to intimidate people. Make people feel good about themselves and you will be the most popular person around.

Check out the box on 'How to keep Friends Happy' (left). Ask yourself if you do those things at least some of the time. If not, now is the time to begin being a better friend.

Finding that soul-mate

Your partner may be a soul-mate but nothing beats having someone who isn't a lover to talk to about everything. If you are lucky enough to have such a person in your life, recognize his or her importance to you and cherish that friendship. You can't conjure up such friends to order. If you follow all the tips in this workshop, however, you will put yourself in line for finding one. Usually when we meet a soul-mate, we know almost instantly. You start talking and never stop, and friendship seems natural from that moment. Nothing is forced, there is no need to try. That kind of closeness is very special. It doesn't mean you will never argue or fight or annoy each other, but it is true deep friendship.

Sometimes your soul-mate is harder to detect – it may even be the person about whom you said, 'I could never be friends with HER!' Underneath that arrogant or perfect or untouchable or superior facade may be the loneliest, but nicest, person around. Never give up on people until you've tried.

Sometimes the best friends come well disguised.

Your Family Matters

Are you lucky enough to have a family. . . Parents, brothers, sisters, children, grandchildren, cousins, uncles, aunts. . . ?

If you are, do you enjoy them and appreciate them enough? Sadly, very many of us don't. For some of us, lack of close family contact is a result of the way we've lived our lives so far. Women now in their late 30s, 40s and early 50s are the first generation of women to realize the true price we paid for the career ethic.

• We moved away from our family home or area to get the education and then the job we wanted.

• One in three of us got divorced and fragmented the family further.

• We maybe had our own children cared for by other people most of the time and don't feel as involved with them now as we would like.

• We were so busy building our careers and our nest-eggs that keeping close contact with family didn't seem so important.

• We had our children later than our forebears did; our own children are having their children late, too – meaning we all have to wait later for grandchildren, nephews, nieces and so on. The result? We've got out of the habit of closeness with family, and, whether we choose to admit it or not, that can lead to loneliness, loss of support, feelings of guilt – but, most importantly, loss of pleasure and loss of a sense of belonging. Of course this isn't true for all of us, but it is true of a surprisingly high number. And for those of us who didn't go that route and do have a family nearby, many of us quite simply take that family for granted. We may even moan about them. Whether you have distant family, fragmented family, or family in proximity you don't appreciate, you may like to think of the millions of people who aren't lucky enough to make those choices. You can make friends, but you can't make family. So why not begin to realize how fortunate you are to have blood relations, and start making friends of them.

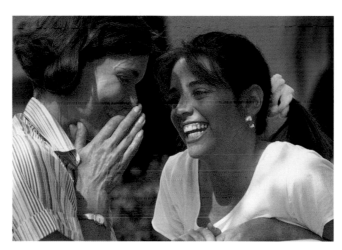

Family checklist

If your family are far away
• phone regularly.
• Write regularly.
• Send and ask for photos, videos, audios to keep in better touch.
• Visit whenever you can. Don't automatically put family last on your list; is work really more important?
• Invite them whenever you can. If you're busy, make sure they help; treat them like family rather than guests.

If your family are near –
• Try to look at their good points rather than their failings.
• Count your blessings.
• Have regular arranged times when you will go and see them/they will come and see you.
• Be on the lookout for relatives who need help. Many are too proud to ask. If you can't help them, who can?
• And don't be too proud yourself to ask for help or admit life isn't going well. Family can be the best shoulders to cry on, even better than friends.

• Try your best to be friends with your ex-husband, and/or your partner's own family.
• Make as much time as you can for your own children and grandchildren. It's time you can never get back and the thing women tend to regret most.

Whether your family are close or away

• Make allowances. Use the same principles in 'How to Keep Friends Happy' box on your relatives.
• If you have an argument, make it up. I have a friend who hasn't seen her only sister for 10 years after an argument about a borrowed outfit. Most family arguments are over quite petty things that aren't worth falling out over.
• Show appreciation. If you can't say it, write it.
• Tell yourself you're lucky. If you want confirmation that you are – talk to most only children, orphans, childless people and you'll soon have your confirmation.

I f you have been with the same partner for a decade or more you may find that some of the early passion, fun and spontaneity have gone from your relationship. It's time to see what (if anything!) can be done.

WORKSHOP 22 RELATIONSHIPS 1 – LONG-TERM LOVE

However slim, fit and energetic you feel towards the end of your 10-week programme, it is hard to feel as fresh and alluring as a 20-year-old on her first date if you are in a long-term relationship that is hovering somewhere between the predictable and the downright stale. There is also perhaps nothing as ageing, mentally, as the realization that your partner thinks you are about as sexy as a pair of old slippers (or vice versa).

But this workshop isn't just about sex, it's about enjoying your partner - and life with your partner - again. That said, if you're a normal woman you will want a reasonable sex-life - all research shows that good sex keeps you young - so let's start from that point.

'Our Sex-life Isn't Great.'

I hate all those articles in women's magazines about how to revive your sex-life with your partner by wearing frilly underwear, strong perfume and cooking his favourite supper by candlelight while wearing little else. Hardly subtle, and hardly ever works. Your partner thinks you have gone slightly crazy and feels embarrassed and you (I hope) feel ridiculous. You'd be better off watching a sexy movie together.

The fact is, however, that if you've been with someone a long time it is almost impossible to recreate the amazing buzz you felt, that spontaneous combustion, of the early months. It may last a few years or so if you're lucky. By the time you hit your tenth wedding anniversary or later, the only way to get that feeling back is to fall in love with someone else.

However, that is not to say you can't enjoy good regular sex. Here's how:

- Make sure you like each other. If one or both of you is filled with underlying resentment or misery you're not really going to want sex. Talk about problems and, if you can't, consider counselling.

- Do enjoyable things together at least some of the time.

- Be nice to him and if he is nice to you, make sure he knows you appreciate it.

- If you are in the menopause and you've gone off sex altogether, see your practitioner – there is plenty you can do, from HRT to natural supplements to pessaries. Don't suffer alone and in silence!

- Take regular time apart from each other. Many couples live in almost constant contact with each other, then wonder why they feel bored.

- Both keep yourselves evolving – Workshop 20 is full of ideas – rather than stagnating. You may find him much sexier if you can see him in a new light. Flirting helps here, too. If he sees you being chatted up by another man he too will see you afresh.

- Keep fit and active and organize your days, both of you (see Workshop 12), so that you aren't exhausted every night when you climb into bed.

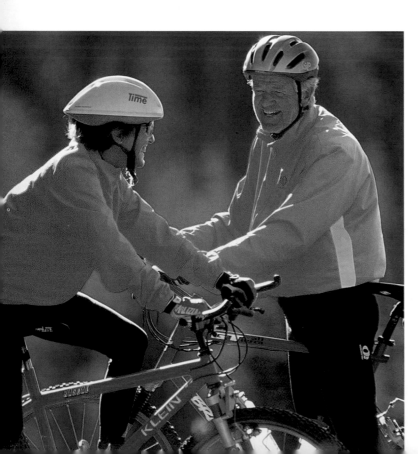

CASE HISTORY

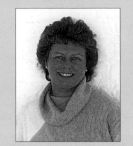

Pamela has been married to her husband Nick for 30 years, and she puts the success of her marriage down to several factors:

'I didn't marry until I was 27, and by that time I had travelled a lot, done and seen plenty, and so was quite ready for the commitment of marriage. Secondly, Nick and I were great friends before we began dating, and I think that is very important – he is still my best friend!

'I think divorce is too easy now, so often I see people split up almost at the first sign of problems; you have to realize that you are two different people and won't always agree; work things out rather than give up easily. With the next partner there are going to be problems too. Nick and I have had our upsets, but you learn to accept your differences.

'And to keep boredom at bay and your marriage alive it is important that you both have your own interests and not spend every moment together. You've also got to keep communicating and not neglect your husband for the children. When they have gone he's the one your going to be stuck with after all!'

Evolving in Your Relationship

I know several women who have divorced attractive kind hard-working generous healthy husbands for no better reason than that, 20 or so years after the wedding, excitement and passion had disappeared. They mostly went off with younger men and some, after 2 or 3 years in a new marriage, are again feeling dissatisfied because the buzz of being 'in love' is already fading. . . even faster than it did the first time.

You have to choose – between making a deep and ever-evolving relationship, or between serial marriage (or partners), or being on your own. For those who manage it, the former is undoubtedly the most rewarding and enriching, and it always amazes me how so many couples split up so lightly after sharing such a lot.

With a successful relationship you simply and gradually replace the things that held you together in your first years – lust, newness, excitement, insularity and so on, with new things – parenting together, friendship, caring, shared interests, a sense of your own history, and so on. You can't have both – but the things that come with time are even better.

Does any of this apply to you? If you're feeling slightly bored and discontent, slightly stale with your relationship and half looking for something better – try, for a change, to see the good things about it.

- Make a list of all the good points about your relationship together.
- Make a list of all the good points about your partner's personality.
- Make a list of all the good points about your life in general. Try also to think through whether your boredom is as much to do with too little going on in the rest of your life as it is to do with your partner.
- Do you have enough platonic friends? (See Workshop 21.)
- Is your job satisfying – or, if you don't have one, should you get one? (See Workshop 18.)
- Is your personal life fulfilling? (See Workshop 21.)

When someone is always around it is easy to stop valuing them, assume they will always be around, and stop trying. However, a good close long relationship is a prize to be cherished. It's so easy to let it go due to carelessness. . . and hard, so hard, to get another. So be as sure as you can be before you tell him it's over.

'Shall I Dump Him?'

We all have the odd day when we could murder our partner – they feel the same. There's no such thing as a perfect relationship all the time. It's all compromise. However, if you're living in a relationship that is making you long-term, chronically unhappy, you don't have to stay. No amount of diet and exercise can take 10 years off your looks if you're being made miserable. Unhappiness is the most ageing emotion of them all, and there is a time to admit defeat and let go – if you stayed for the kids, and now they're grown; if he's had one affair too many; if he's a bully, or violent. . . don't feel sorry for him and stay. Feel sorry for yourself, and take charge of your life.

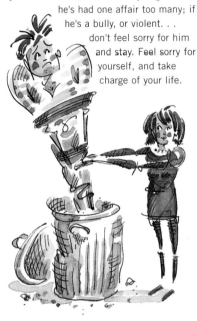

This checklist may help you decide:

1 Is it him who is making you unhappy? Is your own behaviour at fault too? If so, are either of you prepared to try to alter your behaviour? Can you compromise more? Can you settle for less? Do you want to?
2 Does he know how you feel? Have you tried to tell him? Have you succeeded? Would counselling help? (In the UK, try Relate, nationwide, or British Association for Counselling, 01788 578328.)
3 If you still think you should split up, try visualizing your life after the split. If you can make visualizations of your future life and feel positive about it, then you should try. Maybe a 'trial separation' would be possible. If you've lived with someone a long time, an uncertain future can seem almost as bad as a terrible relationship – but you owe it to yourself to try.

S o you're divorced, separated, widowed, or were always too busy to think about a permanent partner. For whatever reason, you're on your own and you're out of practice. But you don't want to be on your own. Quite right. Living alone may be peaceful and blissfully selfish and tidy, but good sex and good love keep you young. Anyway – you don't have to live with him to enjoy both of those. You're old enough and prosperous enough now to need a man only for the pleasures he can offer you. Here you'll find some ideas for finding and keeping that man.

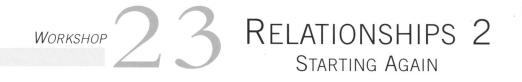

WORKSHOP 23 RELATIONSHIPS 2
STARTING AGAIN

Where Do You look?

I t is often said that if you're looking for a partner, you won't find him, but when you stop looking you will. That is partially true – desperation shows through, is extremely off-putting and should be avoided at all costs. However there is no harm in looking in a relaxed kind of way - to wait and hope to meet someone by chance is likely to involve you in a long wait.

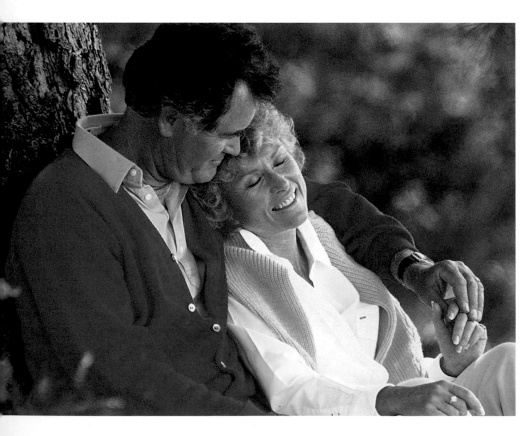

S o where to look? First a list of 'nos' – meeting places that aren't ideal for the newly single mature woman who's out of practice and vulnerable. Some of these 'nos' may be fine for a different sort of person; it's a subjective list.

✗ **NO** to singles bars. They are far too depressing, dodgy and usually make anyone over the age of 25 feel ancient.
✗ **NO** to night clubs. Similarly. A few are OK for older women to go to with a couple of girlfriends, but if you don't choose well you're likely to end your evening feeling very miserable.
✗ **NO** to lonely hearts ads. Whether you put your own ad in the paper or reply to someone else's, it's an extremely soul-destroying way to try to find someone you even like, let alone fancy, and it can be dangerous. If you insist on trying, pick an upmarket paper that is read by people like yourself, and stay very, very cynical.
✗ **NO** to the workplace. Trying to start a relationship at work can be difficult and is rarely wise, whether it's the boss, your assistant or the office 'go-fer'. If you chat him up and get rebuffed, or have a relationship that goes wrong, either way it's going to cause problems.
✗ **NO** to introduction agencies, of the kind where you pay an annual fee and are put in touch with a 'suitable' partner on a one-to-one basis. This may not be a source of

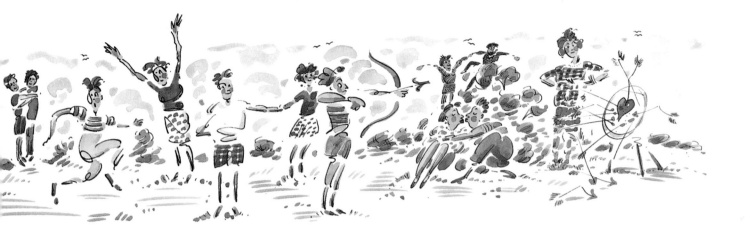

danger, but it is certainly almost as soul-destroying as the lonely hearts ads. After 6 months of being offered 'Mr Rights' who are definitely wrong, your confidence in yourself and in men will be 0%. ✗ **NO** to your best friend's partner. Surprising how often this happens. Follow the tips below, however, and hopefully you won't be that desperate. Nine women out of ten who follow this path lose both their friend and the man, eventually.

That doesn't leave many places to look. Well, yes, it does. The major point to bear in mind is that, once you're over the age of discos and chilling out with your friends on the street, most couples meet in a group situation or while going about normal life. Occasionally it's the instant 'falling in love', but more often you slowly get to love each other. Bearing this in mind let's look at some likely 'yesses'.

✔ **Yes** to private parties, weddings, etc. You have a chance to look stunning and be amongst people you know, so you aren't nervous and always have someone you can talk with. Golden rule - have a maximum of two drinks.
✔ **Yes** with reservations, to blind dates (say, at a dinner party) set up by friends. You should be able to trust your friends to choose, if not someone to whom

you're instantly attracted, then at least someone you like enough to see as a friend.
✔ **Yes** to any hobby or interest club that really does interest you. There's no point joining the local weight-training club in the hope of meeting a hunk if you can't even lift a 1 kilo weight and don't want to - you'll feel and look like an idiot. But if you love walking, or tennis, or photography, or whatever, join a club. Even if you don't find a date there you will make friends who may know other people, etc., etc. And if you're single, you need friends.
✔ **Yes** to an executive friendship club - these are growing fast all over the world as professional people find it harder and harder to meet people through the old-style channels. These clubs are based on weekly meetings, regular events such as theatre visits, dinners, barbecues, picnics, and so on, and are ideal for you as you are within a group of like-minded people, as you would be in a hobby club, but this time they are all single. In the UK, try Nexus, 01237 471704.
✔ **Yes** to activity holidays – some are geared especially for single and/or older people. Ask at your travel agent. If you pick an activity you enjoy – rambling or photography - you don't have to spend hours on your own by the pool feeling lonely. Again, you may not meet a lover but if you spend

your holiday time locked inside your apartment you won't meet one, either – and at least on an activity holiday you'll have fun, which is all part of rehabilitating yourself in the 'outside world', especially if you've been years cloistered with the same partner.

REMEMBER wherever you go – go first looking for companionship and BE friendly yourself. Show your interest in life and in others. If you like someone, let that be a wonderful start. After all, at 20 you may have wanted someone who 'treated you mean' but any sane mature woman will go for kindness and compatibility first and last. The sexiest man in the world isn't going to make you happy for long if you don't like him.

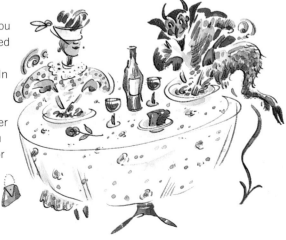

Sex – The New Etiquette

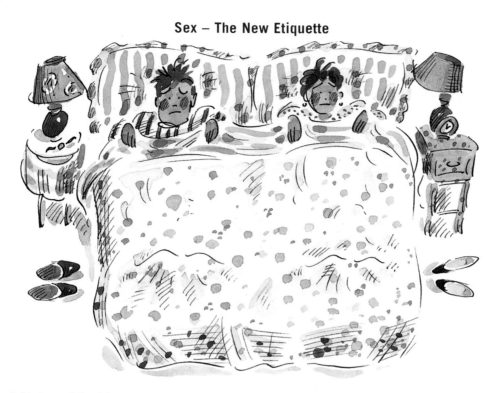

If it is a while (like 10 or 20 years!) since you had sex with anyone new, there are a few things you'll need to know.

• You are allowed to say 'no' at any stage before intercourse; but it is polite to start off as you mean to continue. If you don't want sex, try to make it clear as soon as possible. Even better, before you get into the sexual preliminaries – mouth kissing, for instance – it is better to have had a conversation with him about sex and what you want at the moment. If you have already told him that you'd need to know someone very well before sleeping with him, and he gets heavy on the first date, then he's not being fair and you should say so. It may be that you want sex early in the relationship and he doesn't – not as uncommon as you might think. In that case, it's your turn to be patient.

• You are allowed to ask him to wear a condom and to expect him to have one available and to put it on without complaining. Likewise, you should not take offence if he puts one on before you have a chance to ask him.

• Neither should you take offence if he asks if you've been HIV-tested. You might

like to ask him, too – but it might have been better to get this kind of official business out of the way before you got as far as the bedroom.

• You are not only allowed, but expected, to say what you like done to your body and what you like to do to his; and vice versa. Silence under the duvet is no longer the norm. Neither is turning the lights off – so keep on with the workouts and healthy eating...

• Don't start faking orgasms from night one. If you'd been doing so for years with your previous partner, take this as a great opportunity to change your thinking. Don't fake – talk! What makes a great lover is you telling him what you want and how you're feeling. You can't just assume that even an experienced man knows exactly how to turn you on. Maybe he's been with the same partner for years who's been faking, too – so you can't blame him for getting it wrong. Don't fake – talk! And if you can't talk, perhaps it's too early to be having sex – a piece of advice every mother gives to her teenage daughter, but is true whatever your age.

So Can I Ask Him Out?

Yes, of course you can. However, if you are feeling vulnerable, have never asked a man out in your life before and don't wish to experience what all men have experienced – someone turning you down and making you feel like digging a hole down to the centre of the earth - then it's wise to follow a few precautions:

• Have tickets to something (a football game, the theatre) to flourish in front of him - 'Look, I've just been given these, I know you like football/theatre - do you want to come along?' Yes it's corny, but if he really does like the football game theatre he'll most likely accept unless he can't stand you, in which case you haven't read the signals correctly, and if he wants to turn you down he just has to say, sorry, he's busy that night and you believe him. If it's true, he'll now know you like him and may well ask you to something before long.

• It is also good to invite someone out as if to help you out of a spot. 'Look, I've been invited to a party and I want to go but I'm too scared to go alone as I only know the host. Will you come with me?'

• Always have a purpose in mind for your date apart from the obvious. For instance, it isn't great to just invite him out to dinner at a restaurant or to invite him round to dinner at your place, out of the blue.

• If you're not sure, a daytime date is always the best bet. It seems less predatory to say, 'Come for a picnic with me (and the kids?) in the park if you're not doing anything this weekend!' and if he says no, it's no big deal.

If, in any event, you follow the guidelines on pages 132 and 133 for where to meet someone, by the time you know you want to date him you'll probably not have to worry about how to arrange a date anyway . . . it will all follow on naturally.

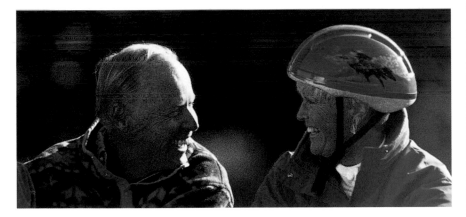

Conquering First Date Nerves

Nervous? Don't worry about it! Just say, 'I feel nervous, I haven't had a date with someone new in a long time.' If he is the kind of man you are going to like, that will be fine. He's probably nervous too. If you meet someone first as a friend or through a common interest, first date nerves won't get a look in because you won't even be sure which was your first date – things will evolve.

Anyhow, if your new date is someone with whom you can be yourself, your nerves will be short-lived. If he isn't – the relationship may never get off the ground, so if he's making you nervous after a few dates – take a look at what you're getting into.

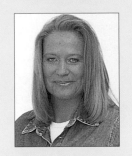

Kay: Having two years ago been through a divorce from the husband with whom she had been for nearly 20 years, Kay was in no rush to meet someone new. 'It has taken me the two years to adjust to living on my own, and to come to terms with what happened,' she says. 'Now, I'm still in no rush, which I think is the best way – but now I can start to say, 'We shall see!'

'I think what you say is right – that if you are totally out of practice at 'dating', the very idea can be daunting – and it is much better to try to build up a network of friends – some of whom may happen to be male. Halfway through the 10-week programme I began a college course 2 days a week, which has been wonderful socially as well. I'm going out to parties now and have met quite a few nice men. And now I am looking better, of course I'm finding a bit more interest. I'm enjoying my freedom now, though – and it will take a special man to change that in the near future.'

*H*ow long is it since you really enjoyed yourself?
Experienced pure, unadulterated pleasure without
a hint of duty or compromise involved?

24 PURE PLEASURE

*I*asked several acquaintances that question and they all had to stop
and think hard to remember such an occasion. Three couldn't
remember one at all, a fact I find very sad.

Nobody could remember the last time they laughed until they
cried; nobody could think of a whole evening spent in pure self-
indulgence. What pleasures there were, were moments or minutes
rather than hours or days. The longer pleasures cited - visits to
the hairdresser by one woman, and a clothes shopping trip
by another - also came with some guilt attached, along
with some unwanted negatives (worrying whether the
hairdresser was going to do the style right;
busy shops, unhelpful assistants and
not finding clothes to fit on the
shopping trip). So, in fact, they
weren't pure pleasure at all.

*W*omen, it seems, are usually
programmed to put everyone
and everything else in life first.
Pleasure comes last, or not at all. Yes,
you say you get pleasure from work
done well, pleasure from seeing your
family enjoy themselves, pleasure
from cooking a terrific meal, passing
an exam. That's pleasure - but it is all
tempered with responsibility or some
other restraining emotion.

What we are bad at is hedonistic
pleasure – pleasure as a beginning
and an end in itself. In other words,
FUN! However great your life is,
however much it is going according

to plan, well organized and without hassle – if you're not having any fun, what's the point?

You need to be carefree, laugh, giggle, indulge yourself – even in small doses – on a regular basis. And you need to do this without guilt. If you feel guilty you're not having fun, and you have no need to feel guilty because pure pleasure is not, ironically, just selfish self-indulgence anyway. There are sound scientifically researched reasons why you should loosen up and enjoy yourself:

• Laughter oxygenates your body, helping you to feel more energetic and sharp.

• Laughter can lower blood pressure but improves both circulation and metabolism.

• Laughter releases endorphins in the body, which are natural pain-killers.

• Laughter boosts the immune system. So laughter may really be 'the best medicine'.

However, you don't have to laugh out loud to benefit from times of pure pleasure. When you are enjoying yourself you are:

Mentally more relaxed – stress levels diminish and so when you get back to your 'responsible' life, you tackle it much better.

Recharging your batteries – a period of real relaxed enjoyment will always help you to carry out tasks with renewed enthusiasm.

Physically more relaxed – facial lines smooth out, digestive problems diminish and after an enjoyable day or evening you are much more likely to get a good night's sleep and thus the effect is an upward spiral.

So let's make Workshop 24 a funshop; let's kill the guilt and let's examine some ways you can be a hedonist and have pure pleasure without a purpose!

Retrogress...

If you've got out of the habit of enjoying yourself you'll need to psyche yourself into it. One of the easiest ways is to think back – maybe even as long ago as your teens; certainly back to your 20s. Think about what you loved to do then, what made you happy; what made you laugh. And now do it again! Have a retro couple of hours. Dig out the old music tapes; look at old photo albums, hire the film or TV series that you loved the most. You may not still think it is all terrific, of course – but it's the feeling of what it was like to be carefree and indulgent that you are trying to get back. Everyone should relish their past and take time to reminisce now and again, anyway. It's soul food.

HEDONISM EXERCISE

Now you make your own list of pleasures large or small. If you are out of practice you may have to think for ages; but the more you do it the easier it becomes. All you have to do now is to enjoy them – but don't forget the rules:

❶
Include nothing except your own, true, real, deep pleasures.

❷
Don't let other people or outside influences dissuade you. *You are as important as anyone else is.*

❸
Don't feel guilty for your pleasure time. Feel guilty if you don't have it!

Progress. . .

Now set aside regular pleasure time and fill it with whatever makes you feel good. *Here are some ideas:*

If you have a few days to spare –
• The holiday you always wanted to take but your partner didn't like.

• A few days in bed with TV, novels, fresh fruit and salads, or whatever food you love and always feel too guilty to eat.

• A few days in bed with your lover.

• A visit to a health farm with as many body massages and facials as you can cram in.

If you have a few hours to spare –
• A visit to the opera/ballet/film/play you've always wanted to see and didn't.

• Watch all the old re-runs of Fawlty Towers or Mr Bean or Ab Fab.

• Who's your favourite comedian? Get his or her tapes and watch them or book a live show.

• Read, read, read (but not heavy educational).

• An evening with your favourite friend just chatting.

• On a perfect day, drop what you're doing and take a slow walk around one of your favourite places.

If you have an hour or less to spare –
• A bath and a glass of champagne.

• A walk round the garden taking time to smell the flowers, see the insects, listen to the birds, soak up the atmosphere. Many people who like gardens work in them all the time but don't take the time to enjoy.

• A sit in a comfy chair in the garden with your eyes shut.

• A phone call to the friend who always makes you laugh.

• A full body massage.

OUR PARTICIPANTS

JUST LOOK AT THEM NOW!

Hilary, 43, finished the 10-week programme weighing 9 stone 7 lb – a 12 pound weight loss, and dead on target. At 5ft 4½ inches, her BMI is now 23.3 and her waist-to-hip ratio just .70.

'The best thing about the programme for me has been the change in my body shape and my fitness. I can swim 30 lengths instead of one, and could probably do more. My legs have never been so slim in my life, and I even like my knees now and am wearing short skirts for the first time. Doing regular exercise has changed so many other things though, too – I have energy, am less lethargic but more relaxed and calmer altogether. My PMS symptoms have improved dramatically, too.

'I enjoyed the diet and I virtually never crave sweet things any more. My skin is better and now I have learnt some make-up tips from Celia I can put them into practice. I love my new hairstyle and so does everyone else – it's so easy to look after.

'The ten week programme was by no means easy all the way through – those early weeks of exercise in particular – but now I'm facing the future with much more confidence, and I feel terrific.'

HILARY 10 WEEKS AGO
She stuck to drab, safe colours, and hadn't changed her hair or make-up in years.

10 WEEKS AGO
Bust 35 in
Waist 29½ in
Hips 37½ in
Thighs 23 in
BMI 25.5
WHR .79
Weight 10 stone 5 lb

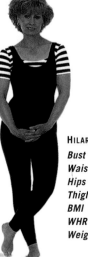

HILARY NOW
Bust 35½ in
Waist 25 in
Hips 35½ in
Thighs 21 in
BMI 23.3
WHR .70
Weight 9 stone 7 lb

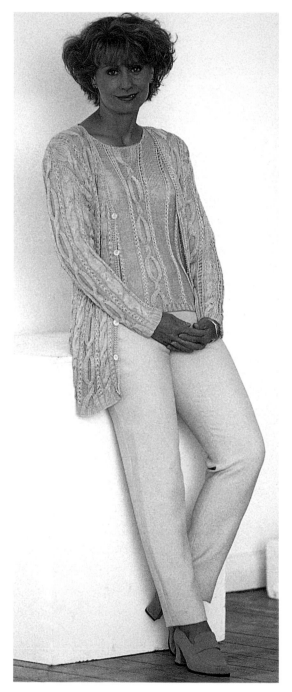

Now Hilary is a total head-turner – and feels much less stressed and more energetic.

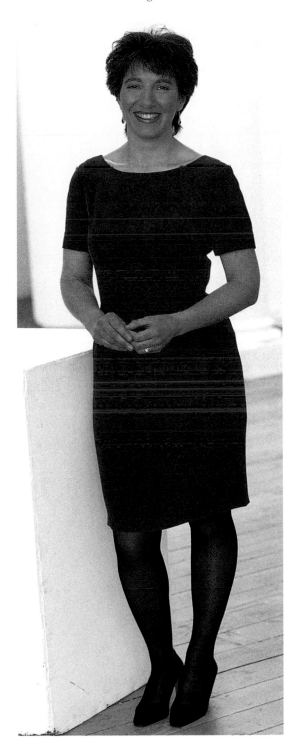

Sue's found her true personality – strong and bright – and an image to match it.

SUE 10 WEEKS AGO
– a dowdy doctor, frightened to find her own style.

When we first met Sue, 39 and 5ft 4 inches, she seemed a shy person for a doctor, almost mouse-like. As the weeks progressed, however, we realized that there was far more to Sue. Her unshakeable determination and strong character began to emerge, and with them, her firm, well-toned, fit new body. Finally, we helped her find her new, bright style to match the rest – and that was it. . . a truly new Sue. 'I enjoyed it all,' she says, 'but particularly having the motivation to do regular exercise – at last I'm as fit as my husband, Steve, now – we've even started going for long cycle rides together. And I needn't feel a bit of a fraud when I tell my patients to exercise and to eat healthily any more!

'Actually, I have very much enjoyed changing my eating habits; I feel better psychologically and physically for it. I think it is due to diet as much as exercise that I feel more energetic throughout the day. I used to suffer from headaches, but even they have diminished. Eating fewer calories was fine – I never felt really hungry or lacking in energy as people often say they do on diets. I ended up losing a stone altogether – slightly lower than the target we set. I shan't lose any more, though, as I don't want to be too slim.'

10 WEEKS AGO
Bust 35½ in
Waist 29½ in
Hips 39½ in
Thighs 22¼ in
BMI 24.7
WHR .75
Weight 9 stone 13 lb

SUE NOW
Bust 32 in
Waist 26 in
Hips 35½ in
Thighs 21½ in
BMI 22.2
WHR .73
Weight 8 stone 13 lb

PAM 10 WEEKS AGO
Pam's look 10 weeks ago was smart, but her hair and clothes were making her 'old before her time'.

Pamela has always taken a pride in her look – buying top-quality clothes, getting her hair done regularly, enjoying good food and enjoying life. However, ten weeks ago, overweight and unfit, with her hair in a typical 50s-plus cut and perm, her dress sense ultra-conservative and her make-up not doing her justice, Pam knew she could do better – she just needed some help.

Now she has lost 13 pounds and taken her BMI and her waist-to-hip ratio within recommended levels – a marvellous achievement. Perhaps more important is the fact that after years of little exercise and a poor level of muscle tone, stamina AND supple-ness – Pam, 5ft 5 inches, is now fitter than she's been in her life, proving that it really IS never too late to start, even if you are on HRT, as she is.

Says Pam, 'I am delighted with the results – so many people have com-mented on how I look. Even my husband likes it – and he hates me to change! My skin and my energy levels are better - and, of course, I can wear so many more clothes now my waist has shrunk. I could hardly believe how much difference the exercise made to my body. At first I couldn't manage more than a few min-utes of exercise without stopping – now I can sail through a whole hour!

'I shall keep up with the exercise and with my healthier eating – doing both means that I can still eat out and entertain more or less when I want to, without having to worry that the pounds will pile back on.'

10 WEEKS AGO
Bust 38½ in
Waist 34½ in
Hips 40 in
Thighs 21½ in
BMI 25.3
WHR .86
Weight 10 stone 7 lb

PAMELA NOW
Bust 37in
Waist 30in
Hips 37½in
Thighs 19in
BMI 23
WHR .80
Weight 9 stone 8 lb

No one can believe Pam is 57 now – she looks more like 37!

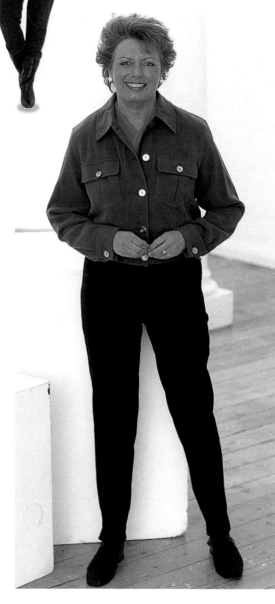

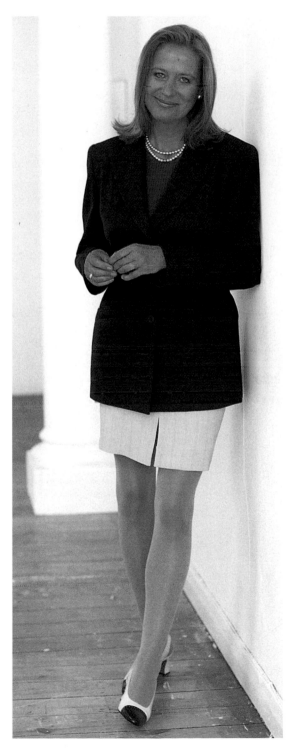

A similar sort of look – but what a difference!

When Kay began the programme, to be honest I wasn't sure that she would come through well. When she tried to exercise, she couldn't follow even basic moves properly and didn't appear to be putting a lot of effort into them either. She actually put on weight the first four weeks because, good for her, she gave up smoking. Then there was a turning point.

I noticed her sweating with effort as she concentrated on the exercise – and Louise and I noticed her figure changing week by week at our weekly weigh- and measure-ins despite the fact that she was losing hardly any weight.

Says Kay, 49 and 5ft 7 inches, 'I began to feel more confident; it was an upward spiral – the more I saw my figure change for the better, the more I was determined to do the exercise. And, as my body improved, so did my self-image and confidence. It's a whole body thing – I used to walk along slowly; now I bounce along! And I feel more supple and lively. With more confidence, the upsets of divorce and redundancy began to seem less threatening, and I could see possibil- ities for me. I realized I could make things hap- pen. I've booked up for swimming lessons, and started training for a new career as a masseuse. I'm chang- ing my life for the better, and I feel great!'

KAY 10 WEEKS AGO
Kay was, in her own words, 'locked in a time warp' with hair and make-up, and was badly in need of advice on dressing for her shape and on updating her wardrobe.

10 WEEKS AGO
Bust 39½ in
Waist 32 in
Hips 38½ in
Thighs 17¼ in
BMI 22.7
WHR .83
Weight 10 stone

KAY NOW
Bust 39 in
Waist 29¼ in
Hips 37 in
Thighs 18½ in
BMI 22.4
WHR .79
Weight 9 stone 12lb

Index

Acknowledgements

The author would like to thank the following people who contributed so much to the book:

Everyone at Quadrille, especially Anne and Alison for their enthusiasm; Lewis Esson for his light touch with my words and for his panic-free professionalism; and Mary Staples for taking on such a task and managing to turn it into something easy on the eye, with a minimum of fuss and no complaints!

The team of expert consultants: personal trainer Louise Taylor who devised the exercise programmes which transformed the participants' bodies in 10 short weeks; Ceril Campbell, style expert, almost as much for the laughs we had as for her marvellous help in preparing Workshops 8 and 9; hair stylist Paul Edmonds, who is a true genius and even made my hair look good; and make-up artist Celia Hunter, whose help with Workshop 6 was invaluable.

Also, Forza Fitness for lending us 'rainy day' fitness equipment for the participants, particularly the amazing Healthrider; Ian Hooton and his team; Jane Turnbull for making it all happen; and my husband Tony, without whom I would have starved while the book evolved.

Most of all I would like to thank the wonderful participants, who did all the hard work while I sat back and watched, and without whom this book would definitely have been the poorer.

The photographs in this book were taken specially by Ian Hooton, except the following:

page 86 Frank Spooner Pictures /Gamma/Y Demeerdt; 93 Camera Press; 96 The Image Bank /Eliane Sulle; 105 Tony Stone Images /David Madison; 108–109 DIAF /H Gyssels; 118 The Image Bank /Bokelberg; 119 Tony Stone Images /Dan Bosler; 120 (right) DIAF /A Feyrier; 121 DIAF /A Feyrier; 125 Tony Stone Images /Howard Grey; 126 The Image Bank /Yellow Dog Productions; 127 Tony Stone Images /Jon Riley; 128 The Image Bank /Eliane Sulle; 130 Robert Harding Picture Library/International Stock; 132 The Image Bank /L D Gordon; 135 Tony Stone Images /Lori Adamski Peek.

The author, the publisher and Ceril Campbell would like to thank the following for supplying items of clothing and accessories for photography:

Azagury, BHS, Carvela, Cox & Power, Dans-Ez International, Debenhams, Dickins & Jones, Dolland & Aitchinson, Episode, Jaeger, Kurt Geiger, Levi's, Roland Cartier, Sign of the Times, Simpson (Piccadilly), Wolford London, Ronit Zilkha

cover: all leotards and tights Dans-Ez International; (group from left to right): orange jacket and coral skirt Episode / shoes Azagury; purple bomber jacket Excursion at Episode/ T-shirt Viyella at Dickins & Jones/ navy lycra trousers J. Taylor at Debenhams / shoes Kurt Geiger; lavender check suit Précis Petite at Dickins & Jones / T-shirt Liz Claibourne at Dickins & Jones / shoes Kurt Geiger; jeans Levi's 611 / boots Kurt Geiger

page 6 suit Louise Kennedy at Simpson / shoes Azagury; 64 spectacles Dolland & Aitchinson; 78 spectacles Dolland & Aitchinson / blue jacket, trousers and striped shirt Petite range at BHS; 79 (top) orange linen jacket and skirt, and coral camisole Episode / shoes Carvela; 79 (bottom left) cream jacket Lolita Lempika from range at Sign of the Times / black trousers Episode / shoes Carvela; 80 (bottom right) shirt, waistcoat, chinos and trainers all at BHS; 81 lime shantung jacket and dress Episode/ shoes Azagury; 82 (right) navy check coat dress Jesiré at Dickins & Jones / shoes Azagury; 82 (left) turquoise cardigan, tunic top and skirt all at Jaeger / shoes Azagury; 85 pale turquoise suit Anne Brooks at Debenhams / shoes Azagury; 84 (bottom) green T-shirt and blue trousers BHS; 84 (right) red silk shift dress Episode/ shoes Azagury; 87 cream-and-black dress Episode/shoes BHS; 88 tweed trouser suit Votre Nom/ silk shirt Episode / shoes BHS; 89 navy jacket and cream striped skirt Epsiode / shoes Roland Cartier; 90 red suit Jesiré at Dickins & Jones / shoes Azagury; 91 striped jacket Episode; 90 navy and red knit dress Country Casuals at Dickins & Jones / shoes Azagury

Please note that the outfits shown in the book may not all be available by the time of publication. There will, however, be similar items available in the credited outlets from the current season's collections by the same designers.